Studies in Acute Heart Failure

To my Wife

Studies in Acute Heart Failure

Ronald D. Bradley

BSc, BS

Consultant Physician, Intensive Care Unit and Consultant Clinical Physiologist, St Thomas's Hospital, London

Edward Arnold

First published 1977
by Edward Arnold (Publishers) Ltd
25 Hill Street, London W1X 8LL

British Library Cataloguing in Publication Data

Bradley, Ronald D
Studies in acute heart failure.
1. Heart failure
I. Title
616.1′2 RC682

ISBN 0-7131-4295-2

Filmset in 'Monophoto' Ehrhardt 11 on 11½ pt by
Richard Clay (The Chaucer Press), Ltd, Bungay, Suffolk
and printed in Great Britain by
Fletcher & Son Ltd, Norwich

Preface

In an age so obsessed with the publication of bewildering quantities of scientific information, there is a need for a concise, cohesive statement of the principles of operation of the central circulation in the clinical state, which, by usage, is referred to as heart failure. This state emerges as a complex of many different conditions, all of which tend to produce a common set of physical signs, but which, when their physiology is understood, are seen to be widely differing states with very different remedies. Out of the course of lectures which are embodied in this book, there sprang some fundamental thoughts about what is, and what is not, heart failure, and the realization that the reflex response of a physician to a raised venous pressure is not always physiologically justifiable.

The principles outlined in the first two chapters, and the examples detailed in the subsequent sections, are intended to help all those who, in the course of their work, manipulate the circulations of their fellow men. The original information which forms the basis of the thesis was obtained in collaboration with Dr B. S. Jenkins, Dr M. A. Branthwaite and Dr J. A. Bell, all of whom shared in the authorship of the ideas which are the mainspring of this brief essay.

RDB

London, 1977

Contents

I

Problem and Hypothesis

This book is the transcription of a set of lectures upon the physiology of circulatory disorders. It is not intended to be comprehensive; rather it is meant to illustrate the principles of operation of the central part of the circulation, its derangement in common clinical disorders, and to leave the reader with a sufficient understanding of the cardiovascular mechanism that he may manipulate the circulation of his patients in a manner which is tailored to their disease pattern.

1.1. The clinical recognition of heart failure

Much of the book is concerned with the physiology of heart failure. Heart failure is recognized clinically as a collection of symptoms and physical signs, of which the most outstanding are breathlessness, effort intolerance, orthopnoea, tachycardia, a raised jugular venous pressure, oedema, basal crepitations and the presence of added heart sounds. The proposition that patients who have heart failure have a raised venous pressure, and that therefore any patient who has a raised venous pressure has heart failure, is neither logically admissible nor physiologically true. The same may be said of all the symptoms and signs listed above, and yet the clinical recognition of heart failure depends upon this illogical assumption. The failure of logic would be of little account were the optimal treatment of all the conditions producing these signs and symptoms the same. Most if not all the symptoms and signs detailed appear in overtransfusion, acute nephritis, acute massive pulmonary embolism and chronic cor-pulmonale. This has led to such patients being treated as if they indeed had heart failure. It will emerge that physiological understanding of these conditions will justify differing therapeutic approaches to the problems. It is not physiologically justifiable to group all these conditions together under the one heading of heart failure and treat them in the same manner.

1.2. The three cartoons (Fig. 1)

The three cartoons are the central theme of this book. They came to be drawn as the result of the death of two patients. Like any cartoons, they prove to be exaggerations of the true state of affairs. They do, however, offer a sensible physiological hypothesis to account for the deaths of these patients.

1.3. The patients who started this train of thought

The first patient was a young haemophiliac aged 17, who proved at post mortem to have a heart which was indistinguishable from normal. He was thought to be suffering from a large retroperitoneal haemorrhage, although ultimately this proved to be small. Over the course of 36 hours 2·5 litres of fresh plasma was transfused with the object of restoring his circulating blood volume, and at the same time, repairing the levels of anti-haemophilic globulin. The pattern of circulatory derangement then presented by this patient appeared to be that of heart failure, inasmuch as his right atrial pressure was grossly raised, he had bilateral pulmonary oedema, and third and fourth heart sounds were clearly audible over both ventricles. The right atrial pressure was measured and found to be 20 mm Hg above the sternal angle. (All pressures reported in this book are related to the sternal angle.) The patient was treated in a manner entirely appropriate to heart failure but failed to improve in any way and went on to die from pulmonary oedema.

Ultimately, as any patient dies his heart must fail, since in death neither ventricle produces any work, irrespective of the height of the filling pressure. Evidence will be presented in Chapter 3 that the equations of performance of both sides of the heart may still be normal in the presence of overtransfusion, at a time when all the signs of heart failure listed in section 1.1 are present.

The second patient, a man of 58, had an abnormal heart, grossly enlarged on a chest x-ray, with third sounds audible over both ventricles. The patient had been demonstrated to have a diminished blood volume following surgery, the measured blood volume being 1·1 litres less than the putative normal blood volume; 250 ml of blood were transfused over the course of 120 minutes, during which time the patient's right atrial pressure rose from 3 to 5 mm Hg. This small increase in right atrial pressure was accompanied by the appearance of dense pulmonary oedema in both lungs and the patient's subsequent death.

1.4. The problem presented by these patients

Here were two patients dying of pulmonary oedema, one with a right atrial pressure of 20 mm Hg and the other with a right atrial pressure of only 5 mm Hg. At post mortem the haemophiliac boy had a normal heart and the other patient severe left ventricular fibrosis due to coronary artery disease. In the first patient the pulmonary oedema appeared only after an enormous rise in right atrial pressure, whereas in the second a trivial rise apparently produced lethal pulmonary oedema.

1.5. The hypothesis

The essence of the hypothesis, constructed to explain the discrepancy, was a forecast of the way in which the normal physiology described in dogs by Sarnoff and Berglund[1] might be distorted in disease. The normal and two of the most interesting distortions are illustrated in Fig. 1. These are the diagrams which have

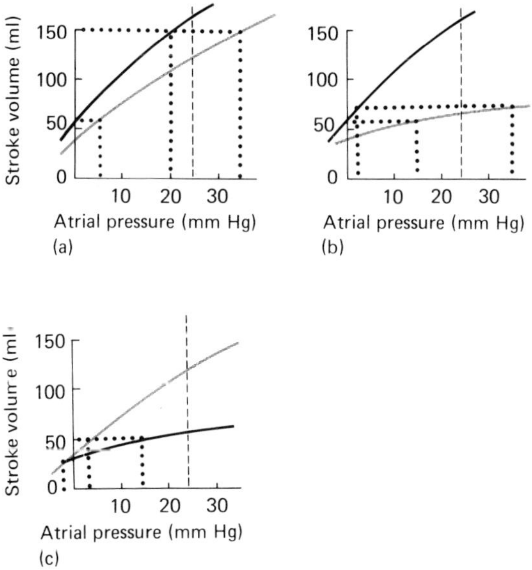

Fig. 1 The three cartoons: (a) normal heart; (b) failing left heart; (c) failing right heart. In each, the stroke volume pumped is plotted on the ordinate, and the right and left atrial pressures on the abscissa. The relation between stroke volume and filling pressure or atrial pressure for the right heart is plotted in black, and for the left heart in grey.

already been referred to as cartoons. In each cartoon the stroke volume of each side of the heart is plotted on the ordinate, and the right and left atrial pressure on the abscissa. The relation between stroke volume and filling pressure or atrial pressure for the right heart is plotted in black and for the left in grey. The first cartoon was drawn in an attempt to explain what had happened to the haemophiliac, the second to account for the observations in the patient with ischaemic heart failure, and the third simply because it was logically inescapable having drawn the first two.

1.6. Values appropriate to a normal at rest

Consider for a moment only the first cartoon, Fig. 1a. If a normal right atrial pressure of 0 mm Hg is applied to the right heart it will project a stroke volume of 60 ml into the pulmonary circulation. The system will only be in balance and the pulmonary blood volume constant if the left heart is pumping an exactly equal stroke volume out of the pulmonary circuit at the other end. The diagram shows that the left heart will do this when the left atrial pressure is 5 mm Hg. These are representative values of those found in a normal patient at rest.

1.7. Suggested values after overtransfusion

If the right atrial pressure is raised to 20 mm Hg by transfusion, the stroke volume of the normal right heart will rise as high as 150 ml. During the course of such a transfusion more blood will be pumped into the pulmonary circulation than the left heart is removing. Some of the increased blood volume occasioned by transfusion of the systemic venous system will thus be redistributed into the pulmonary circulation. This increase in pulmonary blood volume will cause a rise in the pulmonary venous and left atrial pressures. The left atrial pressure will continue to rise with the increasing pulmonary blood volume until the stroke output of the left heart is again equal to that of the right. This will happen according to the diagram (Fig. 1a) when the left atrial pressure reaches 35 mm Hg. This would be an acceptable state of affairs were it not for the height of the left atrial and pulmonary capillary pressures, at which this steady state is achieved, for at this level pulmonary oedema will be generated rapidly.

1.8. Critical value of left atrial pressure at which pulmonary oedema forms

Guyton[2] has shown in dogs that pulmonary oedema occurs once a critical value of left atrial pressure is exceeded. The critical value for dogs with normal serum albumin levels is of the order 24 mm Hg. If the albumin level is half normal, the critical value comes down to 12 mm Hg. The rate of oedema formation depends upon the amount by which the critical value is exceeded.

The lungs will, of course, become stiffer as blood is transferred from the systemic into the pulmonary circulation before the critical value of left atrial pressure is reached; the patient may therefore become breathless before pulmonary oedema appears.

1.9. The second cartoon: a failing left heart

Let us now consider a heart with a severely deranged left ventricle but a normal right ventricle (Fig. 1b). At a filling pressure of 0 mm Hg the normal right heart, as in the first cartoon (Fig. 1a), will pump 60 ml/beat into the pulmonary circulation. The left heart will pump this 60 ml/beat out of the pulmonary circulation but only at the expense of a left atrial pressure of 15 mm Hg. In this state the patient has a normal right-sided filling pressure, in other words a normal central venous pressure, and a normal stroke output from both sides of his heart. The only abnormality is a left atrial pressure of 15 mm Hg, in contradistinction to a left atrial pressure of 5 mm Hg which would obtain, as we have seen, in a normal. In this state the patient may have no signs of heart failure, his venous pressure is normal, his stroke output (and therefore his cardiac output) is normal; the only value which is abnormal is the left atrial pressure of 15 mm Hg, and this is extremely difficult to discern clinically from physical signs. If, however, a history is taken from the patient, it will become clear that he has indeed something wrong with his heart. The patient will give a history of orthopnoea; this occurs because, should he slip down in the bed and lie a little flatter, his right atrial pressure will rise, perhaps only by a trivial amount: 2 mm Hg. This happens because of an alteration in the relative heights of the systemic venous reservoir and the right atrium. The increase in right atrial pressure so engendered raises the stroke output of the right heart from 60 to 75 ml/beat. Inspection of Fig. 1b will show that the left heart can only match this increase in stroke volume with a rise in left atrial pressure from 15 to 35 mm Hg. Again this will cause the rapid generation of pulmonary oedema. The distinctive feature of such patients is the considerable difference in slope between the performance curves of their left and right heart, and it is always true for these patients that small increments in right-sided filling pressure will produce relatively large increases in left-sided filling pressure.

There are many manoeuvres which may bring relief to such a patient; it may be sufficient to sit the patient upright, lowering the effective filling pressure of the right heart. Morphine, aminophylline, diuretics or a small venesection are all effective, either because they are venodilators or because they reduce the circulating volume to produce a small fall in right atrial pressure, which need only be minor to produce a large fall in left atrial pressure and pulmonary capillary pressure.

1.10. The reason that treatment for heart failure is ineffective in overtransfusion

If the same measures which are well known to cure left heart failure are applied to a patient suffering from overtransfusion, reference to the first cartoon (Fig. 1a) will show that, because the performance curves are more nearly parallel, a small fall in right atrial pressure will produce only a small fall in left atrial pressure and pulmonary capillary pressure. This is inadequate to reverse the situation.

Because morphine, aminophylline and diuretics produce only a modest fall in right atrial pressure, an overtransfused patient with a normal heart who is in danger of death from pulmonary oedema should be treated by a venesection of the order of 1·5 litres in volume. The blood which is removed from the circulation may subsequently be returned following the removal of a sufficient volume of fluid from the patient, either through the kidneys or by dialysis.

1.11. A failing right heart in the presence of a normal left heart

The third cartoon (Fig. 1c) was constructed from an admixture of hypothetical possibility and logical necessity. It seemed possible that such a state of affairs might exist, and important to speculate upon the logical consequences of such an arrangement.

It will appear eventually that although this configuration does occur in nature, it comes about as a result of an increased load upon the right heart rather than its failure, although failure was the thought behind the construction of the hypothesis.

In this case, a right atrial pressure of 0 mm Hg produces a stroke volume of only 30 ml/beat from the right ventricle. The matching stroke volume is produced by the normal left ventricle with a left atrial pressure of −2 mm Hg. It seemed possible that elevation of the right atrial pressure to very high levels would raise the stroke volume of the right heart. In Fig. 1c if the right atrial pressure is raised to 15 mm Hg, the right ventricular stroke output rises to 50 ml/beat, which can be matched by the left heart with a left atrial pressure of 3 mm Hg, a level far remote from those which would produce pulmonary oedema, and the stroke volume of the heart has been considerably increased.

1.12. The performance curves and the therapeutic objective

The performance curves of the two sides of the heart as described in these cartoons provide a structure for understanding major abnormalities of the central circulation. Implicit in their understanding is an answer to such problems as the provision of the best possible cardiac output, where its level is critically low, without causing pulmonary oedema. The measurement, or the reasoned assessment, of the pattern of the performance curves will enable treatment to be tailored to the individual patient's pattern of derangement.

2

The Theoretical Background

If the abnormal circulation is to be manipulated intelligently, it is necessary to understand the factors which determine the shape of the performance curves that have been considered, and the relation of the curves to those parts of the circulation which lead into and out of each side of the heart.

The Mechanism—1

2.1. The inflow to the right heart; the venous return

There are certain intellectual difficulties connected with the concept of venous return, which disappear if the student will think in terms of venous pressure. The proposition that the venous return controls the cardiac output, and the idea that the heart can only pump out such blood as has been returned to it, have both been the source of unnecessary confusion. Essentially the heart is the only important pump causing the blood to circulate, and moment to moment alterations in cardiac output are brought about by variation of the performance of the pump.

In a closed circulation the cardiac output and the venous return must ultimately be equal, and because they are mathematically equal, it is unhelpful to think of the one controlling the other.

An example which perhaps illustrates most clearly the fallacy of thinking in terms of venous return controlling cardiac output is the effect of transfusion (in this case the circulation is no longer closed) upon a heart which is failing sufficiently severely to have a constant low stroke output, whatever its filling pressure. The venous return to the heart will be increased by the volume by which the heart dilates in the face of an increasing filling pressure, but the stroke volume and heart rate will not change, and therefore the cardiac output will not change in spite of an alteration in venous return.

2.2 The systemic venous capacity bed

In a normal man the systemic venous capacity bed contains 3·5 l of the total 5 l blood volume. If the volume which it contains is held constant, and the tone of the walls of the compartment (systemic venous tone) increases, then the central venous pressure or right atrial pressure must rise. If the tone diminishes the right atrial pressure must fall.

This action and its effect upon the filling of the right heart are illustrated by Fig. 2. The diagram shows that the volume of blood in the systemic venous capacity bed and the right heart is distributed

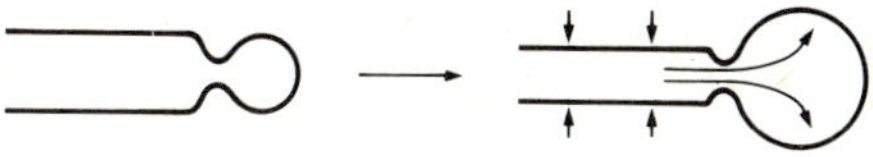

Fig. 2 An increase in venous tone will cause a shift of blood out of the systemic capacity bed into the right heart, which will distend.

between these two compartments in accordance with their relative compliances.

The effect of an increase in venous tone is illustrated; it will cause a shift of blood out of the systemic venous capacity bed into the right heart, which will distend accordingly. Lest it be thought that this shift represents the increase in venous return to the heart which will eventually be translated into an increase in stroke output, let it be said at once that the increase in stroke volume which it will engender will depend upon the state of contractility of the right heart. Thus if, by increasing the venous tone, 10 ml of blood are displaced from the venous system into the right heart, the latter may respond by an insignificant increase in stroke volume of less than 1 ml per beat, or with a much larger increase in stroke volume depending upon its state. It is the behaviour of the heart which will determine the change in stroke output in response to a change in its filling.

2.3. The influence of varying the volume in the capacity bed

If the venous tone could be held constant and the volume of blood in the

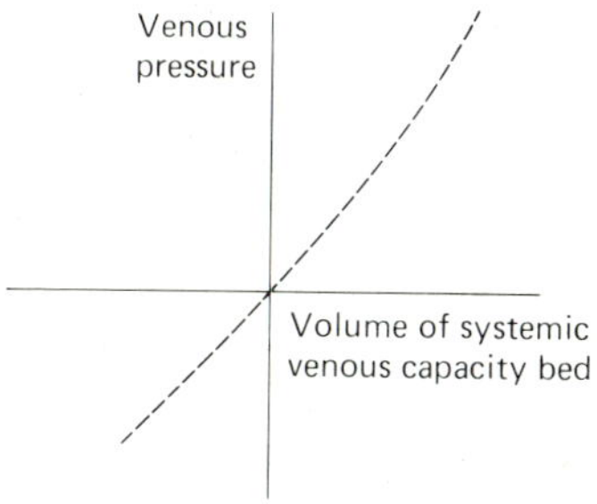

Fig. 3 The relation between venous pressure and the volume of blood in the systemic venous capacity bed, under conditions of constant venous tone.

venous capacity bed varied, the right atrial pressure would rise and fall in a predictable way as the volume was increased and decreased. This idea is illustrated in Fig. 3 which is in effect the compliance diagram of the combined venous capacity bed and right heart in diastole.

2.4. Lines of constant venous tone

The relation plotted in Fig. 3 is an imaginary concept, for it is a line representing the relation between the volume contained by the venous capacity bed and the right atrial pressure under conditions of constant venous tone. Such a line could be called an 'isophleb'. There are of course an infinite number of isophlebs, each one representing a line of constant venous tone, as shown in Fig. 4.

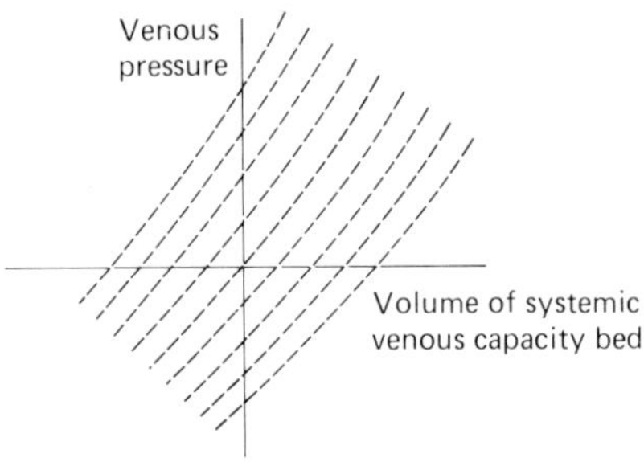

Fig. 4 There are an infinite number of lines (isophlebs) relating venous pressure to volume contained by the capacity bed, each at constant venous tone.

2.5. The systemic venous capacity bed and haemorrhage

Although isophlebs are an imaginary concept (because it is impossible experimentally to keep the venous tone constant whilst altering the volume of blood in the capacity bed), they provide an ordered background against which events which are capable of measurement may be viewed.

Consider haemorrhage in these terms. As blood is removed from a normal circulation, the initial fall in right atrial pressure is small, but as the haemorrhage continues, the fall in right atrial pressure becomes greater in relation to the volume removed. In Fig. 5 it will be seen that as the first aliquot of blood is removed (A to B), the right atrial pressure drops by a small amount; the removal of further aliquots (B to C, C to D and D to E) produces successively greater decrements in right atrial pressure until it reaches the lowest values seen in patients suffering from acute haemorrhage, in the region of −10 mm Hg.

The relation ABCDE is convex upward because the walls of the capacity bed are not simply behaving as an elastic material. (Over this range of volume change, the changes in radius or circumference of the vascular bed are nearly linear with change in volume. If the walls were a perfect elastic material then the fall in right atrial pressure would be approximately linear with volume.) The observed shape can only be explained by a rise in venous tone.

The increase in venous tone which occurs during haemorrhage can be observed clinically. In the context of a patient in a warm hospital bed, as the venous system constricts the superficial veins of the feet will constrict first, then the hand and arm veins disappear, and finally the venules of the face constrict producing intense facial pallor. These are the clinical observations which may be noted as the patient progresses down the line ABCD in Fig. 5.

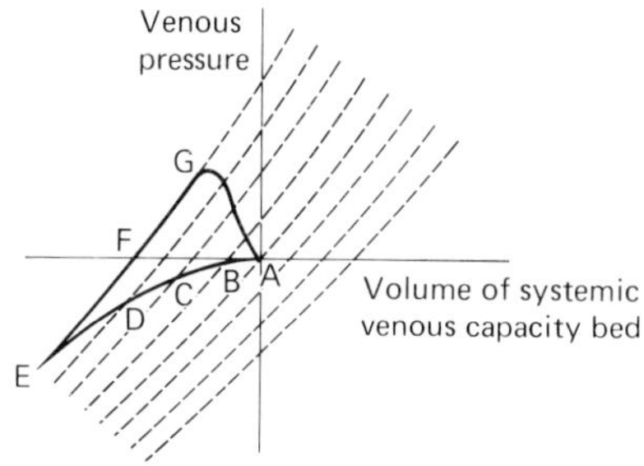

Fig. 5 As blood is removed from the circulation, the venous pressure falls little initially, but later more steeply, as the patient proceeds to lines of greater venous tone. With retransfusion the patient should follow the path EDCBA; return via EFGA may produce pulmonary oedema.

2.6. Transfusion of the exsanguinated, and why there is sometimes not enough space for the volume which has been lost

Transfusion of a patient who has sustained sufficient blood loss to arrive at the point E in Fig. 5 may be entirely uneventful. As the blood which has been lost is replaced, the right atrial pressure may steadily return to normal and the patient's venous system may be observed to dilate in the reverse order to which it constricted, return to the point A being signalled by a normal right atrial pressure and dilated foot veins.

There are a number of changes which may take place whilst the patient is at E, which will frustrate this simple return to normality with transfusion. At E the patient has a right atrial pressure of −10 mm Hg, and as a consequence will have an inadequate cardiac output, and very poor coronary perfusion. If this state of affairs continues for any length of time, it will bring in its train metabolic acidosis, a fall in body temperature, myocardial damage and, in some cases, the low flow through the lungs produces mismatch of perfusion and ventilation, and therefore hypoxia. All or any of these factors cause the venous tone to remain high when the missing blood volume is restored. Because the venous system does not dilate, restoration of only half the volume which was lost, brings the right atrial pressure back to normal (the point F in Fig. 5). If transfusion of the volume, which is known to have been lost, continues, the right atrial pressure rises to values above normal (G in Fig. 5). Most commonly this high right atrial pressure restores the cardiac output. This will allow adequate tissue perfusion with reversal of the metabolic acidosis, rewarming of the patient and the restoration of an effective coronary flow. The re-establishment of the cardiac output will also abolish the ventilation perfusion defect in the lungs. The venous system then dilates and the patient is restored to normality (point A in Fig. 5). Unless the patient's venous pressure has been measured, it is unlikely that it will be known by which pathway he has been restored to point A. There are a number of patients for whom the path EFG is potentially lethal. Patients whose right and left hearts are related in the manner described in the second cartoon (Fig. 1b) may die of pulmonary oedema if their venous capacity bed fails to dilate. It should be noted that they may die of overtransfusion before the volume of blood, which they are known to have lost, has been replaced.

The concept is a simple one and depends upon the fact that the vascular bed has undergone a considerable reflex volume change, and will no longer hold the volume of blood which it previously accommodated.

2.7. The safe control of transfusion

If, as a patient is transfused, his venous system shows no evidence of dilating by the time that the right atrial pressure has risen to −2 mm Hg, the matter should be investigated. Acidaemia, hypoxia, hypothermia and pain are all readily treatable causes of a sustained high venous tone. Myocardial damage probably keeps the venous tone high by limiting the cardiac output in spite of the restoration of the filling pressure. This can be offset by inotropic stimulation (causing the heart to do more work at the same filling pressure), although if there is ECG evidence of ischaemia, it may be better to wait upon the results of the correction of all the other factors, and the passage of time.

If the patient's heart is normal, restoration of the right atrial pressure to a normal level will produce a normal cardiac output.

If the patient has the abnormality characterized by the second cartoon, elevation of the right atrial pressure above normal may produce pulmonary oedema.

If the patient suffers from the anomaly described in the third cartoon (Fig. 1c), then it may be desirable to raise his right atrial pressure to levels above normal, but such a patient would be unlikely to survive an extensive haemorrhage, because low atrial pressures are associated in this instance with insupportably low levels of cardiac output.

It is only in most unusual circumstances, therefore, that in the treatment of haemorrhage the right atrial pressure should be brought above normal. The observations necessary for control and understanding of volume replacement are the right atrial pressure and the state of constriction or dilatation of the peripheral veins.

Control of transfusion by measurement, either of the volume lost or of the volume remaining in the circulation, may be misleading or even dangerous.

Whilst still concerned with the behaviour of the venous capacity bed, the reader may wish to consider the implications of overexpansion of the circulating volume in terms of Fig. 5, and of the situation in barbiturate intoxication in which the venous tone is fixed and lower than normal, and the patient may also be oligaemic because of dehydration.

2.8. Dynamic influences on right atrial pressure

The determinants of right atrial pressure so far considered—the tone of, and volume contained by, the capacity bed—might be called 'static' determinants of filling pressure to the right heart. They are static in the sense that a given volume change or tone change would have the same influence on filling pressure, whether the flow through the system were 2 l/min, 20 l/min, or if there were no flow at all.

The dynamic determinant of atrial pressure is illustrated with a simple model of a closed circulation containing a pump and a resistance (Fig. 6). When the pump is adjusted so that it pumps 5 l/min around the circuit, it does so by generating a positive pressure on its output side, and a negative pressure on the input side. The pressure levels generated are illustrated by the levels +5 and −5 in Fig. 6. In order to achieve double the flow rate in an ideal system, the pressure difference generated by the pump would require to double (+10 and −10 in Fig. 6). If the flow rate were to be cut to 2 l/min, the pressure on the output side would fall and on the input side would rise (+2 and −2 in Fig. 6). In this simple system the pressure on the input side of the pump represents the pump's ability to suck, or its inability to do so as it fails.

It is probably from an analogy such as this that misconceptions concerning the rising venous pressure in heart failure, indeed the very term 'congestive' heart failure, arise.

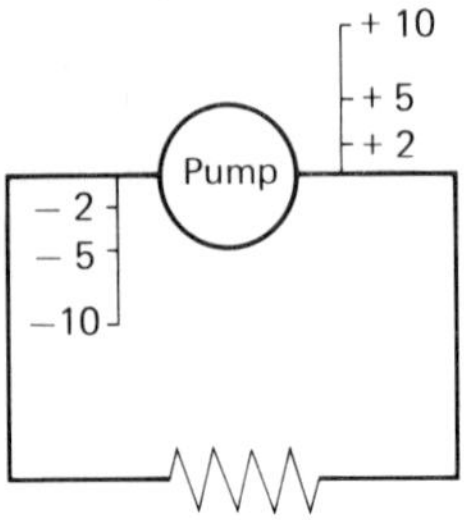

Fig. 6 Dynamic determinants of filling pressure; the tractive or sucking effect of the pump varies with flow rate.

The venous pressure does not rise in heart failure because the blood is being 'dammed back' by an inadequate heart. It rises because of a reflex increase in venous tone, and an increase in the volume contained by the capacity bed. The static determinants of filling pressure preponderate so greatly over the dynamic 'suction' produced by the right ventricle, that the latter phenomenon is extremely difficult to demonstrate. The wall of the right ventricle is unlikely to be sufficiently stiff to produce an important tractive effect during diastole.

The Mechanism—2

2.9. The heart

The two sides of the heart are arranged as pumps in series. The central theme of this book is the absolute necessity of considering the operation of both of these pumps in any assessment of circulatory derangements.

Initially the behaviour of a single pump must be considered, and as the principles of operation of both sides are similar, the ensuing description can be taken to apply to both left and right heart.

2.10. Operating characteristics

In a constant state of 'contractility', any chamber of the heart will show a relation between the pressure to which it is filled, and the work that it will generate at each beat. This is one way of defining contractility. The resulting equation of stroke work versus filling pressure is probably best called a function curve. The stroke work throughout this text is defined as (mean output pressure minus mean input pressure) × stroke volume.

2.11. Function curves and the fundamentals upon which they depend

As Fig. 7 shows, the left ventricle produces very much greater amounts of work than the right ventricle or the atria in relation to filling pressure. These function curves are the product of two more

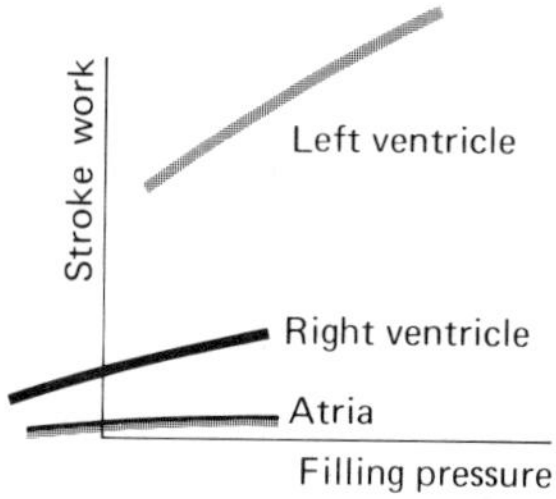

Fig. 7 Function curves. The relation between filling pressure and work produced per beat for each chamber.

fundamental relations. The first relation is that between filling pressure and fibre length of the contractile elements in the chamber wall at the end of diastole (Fig. 8). This is the compliance equation of the chamber, or its 'stretchability' at the end of diastole. The second, that between the fibre length achieved just before contraction occurs and the work generated by that contraction (Fig. 9), is the property of muscle first described by Fick [3] and later by A. V. Hill.[4] The original description referred to striated muscle but the same truth has been demonstrated for cardiac muscle. In the physiological range the active tension, or work generated by the muscle, is linearly related to the length to which the muscle is stretched before contraction is initiated. The degree to which the muscle is stretched

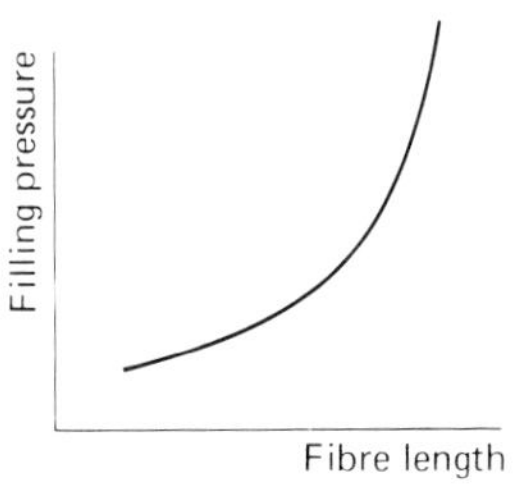

Fig. 8 The compliance or 'stretchability' of the chamber at the end of diastole.

before it is stimulated to contract is variously referred to as the preload or resting tension, but clearly, in the case of heart muscle, any measure of fibre length could be used. End diastolic circumference or radius would be appropriate.

If the common term of fibre length is taken out of these two equations, then work produced is related directly to filling pressure—the function curve. This derivation of the function curve from the two more fundamental characteristics is important because the distortion of the function curve which occurs in ventricular failure may be a distortion of either or both of these two fundamental relations.

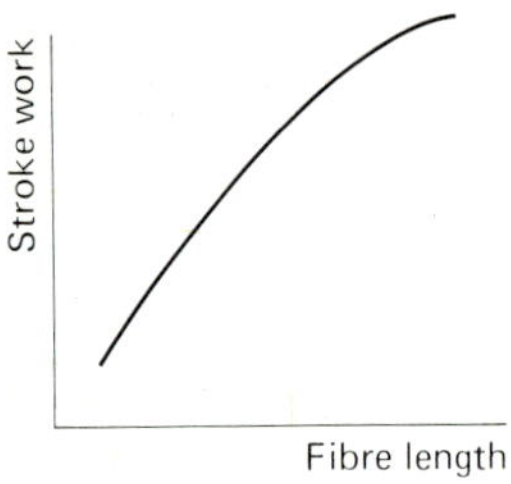

Fig. 9 Active tension, or work generated, related to the length to which the muscle is stretched before contraction is initiated.

2.12. The A. V. Hill relation in heart failure

Either necrosis of a proportion of the contractile elements, as happens in acute myocardial infarction, or dysfunction of all the contractile elements due to acute metabolic changes such as hypoxia, acidaemia or hyperkalaemia, has a depressant effect upon the work generated in relation to fibre length. With increasing dysfunction the slope of the equation decreases, in physiological terms, less work is produced by a given fibre length, and an increase in fibre length produces a smaller increase in work. This change has an exactly similar effect upon the function curve, which becomes flatter.

2.13. The diastolic compliance curve

The diastolic compliance curve has two principal slopes (see Fig. 8). The shallower represents the stretching of relatively elastic elements, predominantly in the contractile mechanism, in the ventricular wall. These stretch considerably with a modest rise in filling pressure. At the inflexion of the curve, a change takes place, and fibrous elements in the wall begin to take up the strain.[5] Because their resistance to elongation is much greater than that of the elastic elements, any further filling of the ventricle can only be obtained by very considerable elevation of the filling pressure.

2.14. Hooke's law and the compliance curve

An elastic material will lengthen and shorten predictably as tension is applied to it and released; but once a certain value of tension is exceeded, the material will stretch permanently, and will then have a different equation of tension versus length. This is shown graphically in Fig. 10. If the elastic and fibrous scaffold elements of the

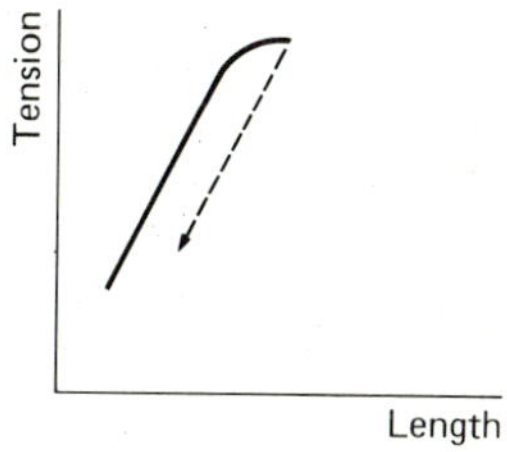

Fig. 10 An elastic material lengthens predictably with increasing tension, but one overstretched moves to a different equation of tension versus length.

ventricular wall are overstretched in this fashion, the compliance curve is shifted to the right in the manner shown in Fig. 11.

A shift of the curve to the right infers that at any given filling pressure, the fibre length will be greater, and a greater fibre length should produce more work, but this is not so, a ventricle which has been overstretched does not produce more work than the normal at a given filling pressure. Other changes have taken place.

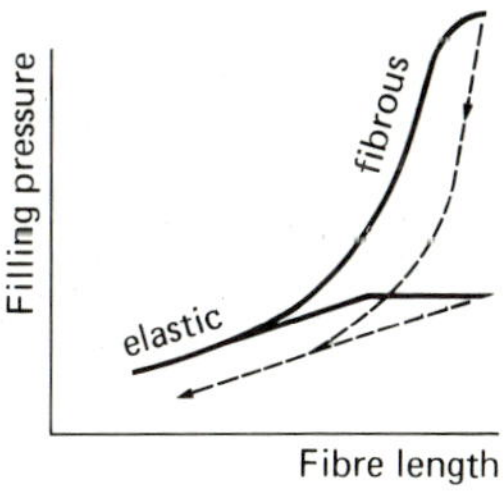

Fig. 11 If the elastic and fibrous elements of the ventricular wall are overstretched, the compliance curve is shifted to the right.

2.15. The relation of Z band to Z band distance and filling pressure in the overstretched ventricle

It has been shown by rapid fixation of both normal and dilated ventricles at known filling pressures[6] that the compliance curve shifts to the right in a dilated, overstretched ventricle, if the equation has been plotted as filling pressure related to a macroscopic measure of chamber size such as circumference or radius. If instead, the microscopic length of the contractile units, that is the Z band to Z band distances, is used as the scale on the abscissa, then the scale shifts to the right with the curve, as is shown in Fig. 12.

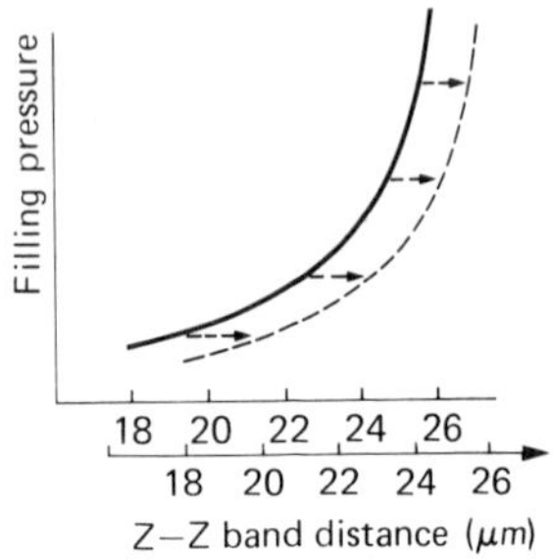

Fig. 12 If Z–Z band distance is used in place of fibre length, the scale on the abscissa moves to the right with the equation.

It is possible to suggest diagrammatically an arrangement in which the gross fibre length could be increased without alteration in the Z band to Z band distance.[7]

Although the Z band to Z band distances in Fig. 13 are the same in both (a) and (b), the gross length of the same number of units is

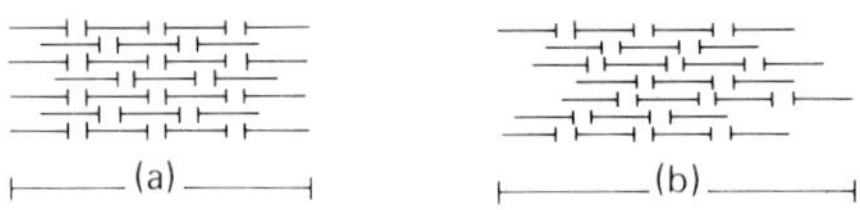

Fig. 13 The contractile units are stretched to the same length in both (a) and (b), but the gross length of (b) is greater, because slipping has occurred between the elements.

greater in (b) because the muscle units have slipped upon one another. It is immaterial to the argument whether or not the muscle fibres have altered their geometrical arrangement in this or some other way. It is also immaterial that the same filling pressure applied to a ventricle of larger radius will produce a larger resting tension or preloading tension in the wall (Laplace's law and the dilating ventricle will be considered in section 2.16). It is known experimentally that the relation between filling pressure and Z band interval is unchanged when the ventricle is overstretched.[6] The active tension generated therefore by contraction of the muscle units in the wall should be the same at the same filling pressure. (This argument neglects thinning of the wall which must take place if the same muscle mass encompasses a larger chamber.)

2.16. Laplace's law and the dilating ventricle

Laplace's law in its simplest form relates the tension in the wall of a sphere of notional wall thickness to the radius of the sphere and the pressure within it. The law may be stated thus:

$$p = \frac{2T}{r}$$

Where p is the pressure within the sphere, r its radius and T the wall tension. (The relevance of this law to the performance of the heart was pointed out in 1892.[8])

Applied as stated to the problem of a dilating ventricle, if the tension generated in the wall is constant, and the radius doubled, the pressure generated within the ventricle will be halved. Because the ventricle is not a sphere and has a wall of finite thickness, the ratio by which the pressure is reduced if the radius is doubled lies between two-thirds and three-quarters.[9] As already stated, if the ventricle dilates and the muscle mass comprising the wall does not alter, then the wall will be thinner, and this will reduce the active tension generated.

These effects summate so that dilatation of a ventricle impairs its capacity to generate pressure grossly. This impairment has the same effect upon the function curve as a defect of the contracting elements.

2.17. The two depressants are usually mixed

In most instances of ventricular failure, the defect in the contracting elements and the increasing radius are both present. The proportion of their responsibility for depression of the function curve varies.

A patient who has just suffered his first episode of myocardial infarction may have ventricles of normal size, and yet have a major disturbance of myocardial function due to death of a proportion of the contracting elements and metabolic disturbance of many others.

At the other end of the spectrum, there are patients whose ventricles have been subjected to an afterload for a long period of time. (An afterload is the added resistance to contraction which bears upon a muscle only after it has begun to shorten—in the case of the heart a load which only acts upon the ventricle after the opening of the aortic or pulmonary valve, for example a high systemic or pulmonary vascular resistance.) In such a ventricle the contractile elements provide a greater than normal tension because of hypertrophy of the ventricular wall. These patients nevertheless have gross depression of their ventricular function curves, because of the increase in ventricular chamber size which follows overstretching of the wall.

2.18. Inotropic agents and the function curve

An inotropic agent, by definition, moves the function curve upward and to the left. It causes the heart to do more work at any given filling pressure. This means that such agents have an exactly opposite effect to ventricular failure upon the function curve.

The substances which have this activity (digoxin and all the cardiac glycosides, isoprenaline, adrenaline, glucagon, salbutamol, dopamine, dobutamine and electrolyte changes having the same effect—hypokalaemia, hypercalcaemia, correction of the pH toward normal) are all appropriate therapeutic agents if the mainspring of the patient's disorder depends upon depression of the curve. If, on the other hand, the principal fault is a disturbance of the relation between the slopes of the equations for the two sides of the heart, these drugs will lift both equations but not alter the ratio of their slopes (see section 4.4).

2.19. Drugs known to depress the function curve

There are many drugs which are well known to exert a depressant effect—β-blockers, quinidine and procainamide. There are many others whose activity in this respect is very much less well known—a number of antibiotics including chloramphenicol and streptomycin,[10] the hypnotic methaqualone, hyperkalaemia, acidosis, hypocalcaemia and hyponatraemia, all have depressant activity. There are many other commonly used drugs, such as morphine, for which the evidence is inadequate. Morphine is frequently used in situations involving critical depression of the function curves by disease, and may, therefore, be undesirable in these circumstances.

2.20. The function curve and an afterload

The function curve of a normal ventricle subjected to an increase in afterload will move upward and to the left.[11] In animals this effect has been demonstrated to be independent of sympathetic or other reflex activity, and to be an intrinsic response of the muscle. It is probable that a failing ventricle does not respond as well as a normal to the imposition of an afterload. Reduction of the afterload in animals produces depression of the function curve, without diminution of the flows in the system because the decrease in ventricular work matches the fall in vascular resistance.

Logically, if a failing heart responds to an increase in afterload with a smaller than normal rise in the function curve, then the

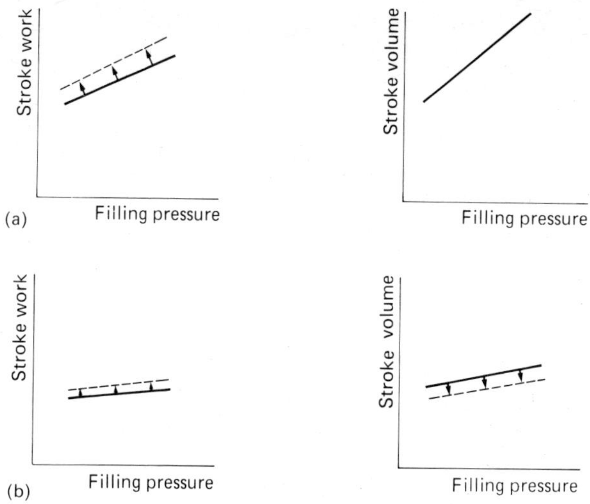

Fig. 14(a) The response of a normal heart to an increased afterload—an elevation of the stroke work equation—allows the equation of stroke volume in relation to filling pressure to remain unaltered in the face of the increased resistance to ejection. Fig. 14(b) The diminished response of the failing heart to the same afterload causes depression of the stroke volume equation. Theoretically therefore removal of an afterload from a failing heart should cause the stroke volume equation to move upward and to the left.

removal of that afterload should occasion a smaller fall in stroke work than would match the resistance change, and ought, therefore, to produce an increase in stroke volume (see Fig. 14). This is the theoretical basis for the current assessments of controlled vasodilatation in situations such as myocardial infarction with severe pump failure. The clinical results of administration of drugs which diminish the afterload proved not to be in accord with the theoretical expectation (see Section 4.17).

The Mechanism—3

Understanding of a clinical circulatory problem, sufficient to allow its intelligent manipulation, requires an analysis of its effects upon all the components of the central circulation. The components whose individual characteristics have already been described, interact continuously so that it is impossible to alter the behaviour of one component without altering the others.

2.21. The components and their interaction

The venous tone, and the volume of blood in the systemic venous capacity bed, determine the filling pressure of the right heart. This value of filling pressure, together with the function curve of the right heart, will determine the stroke work generated. The work generated by the right heart on the one hand, and the resistance into which it empties on the other, control the volume which will be pumped at each beat. This last step, in which the resultant of work produced and the resistance into which it is directed determine the volume pumped, brings the performance equation into the terms which were used in the cartoons, Fig. 1 (stroke volume plotted against filling pressure). This linked chain of events is illustrated in Fig. 15.

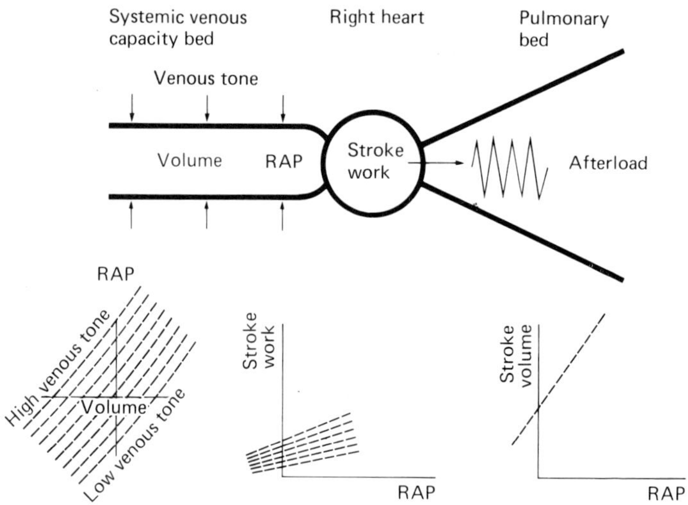

Fig. 15 The venous tone and the volume contained by the systemic venous capacity bed determine the right atrial pressure (RAP), which, with the equation of contractility of the right heart, defines the stroke work which will be generated. The stroke volume delivered into the pulmonary circulation is the resultant of the stroke work and the resistance offered by the pulmonary bed.

The performance of the left heart is determined in an exactly similar fashion. The pulmonary venous capacity bed has a very much smaller volume than the systemic, and its compliance is also less, as is the compliance of the ventricle which it fills. The work generated by the left ventricle, and the resistance into which it empties, are both much greater than the values for the right heart. The principles of operation are identical to those of the right heart and are illustrated in Fig. 16.

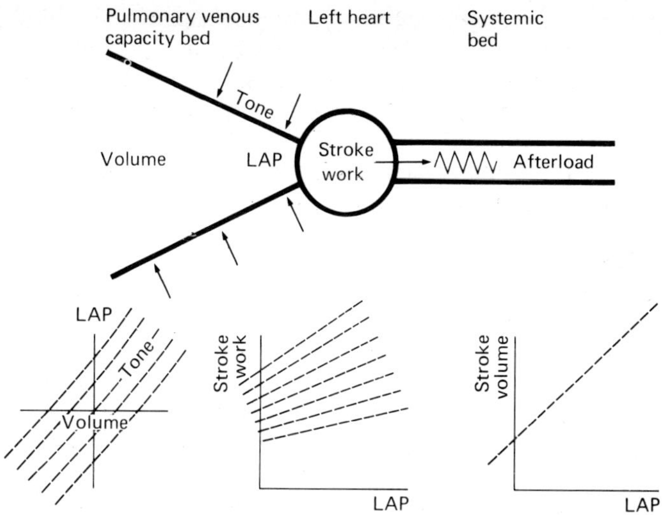

Fig. 16 The pulmonary venous tone and the volume contained by the pulmonary bed determine the left atrial pressure (LAP), which, with the equation of contractility of the left heart, defines the stroke work which will be generated. The stroke volume delivered into the systemic circulation is the resultant of the stroke work and the resistance offered by the systemic bed. The two systems (Figs. 15 and 16) are inexorably locked together by the necessity that the stroke volume pumped by the two sides of the heart must be equal.

2.22. The interlocking of the left and right heart

The two systems are inexorably locked together by the necessity that, in a closed system, the stroke volume pumped by the two sides of the heart must be equal. If the stroke volume of the right heart exceeds that of the left, then each time the heart beats there will be a net transfer of blood out of the systemic into the pulmonary circulation. This transfer will continue beat by beat until the volume of blood in the pulmonary venous capacity bed, and with it the filling pressure of the left heart, has risen to a level which will cause the stroke volume of the left heart to equal that of the right.

If, instead, the stroke volume of the left heart exceeds that of the right, then the net transfer of volume will be out of the pulmonary into the systemic bed, and the filling pressure of the left heart will fall until its output matches that of the right.

The details of the adjustment are a little more complex than this, for with inequality of output, and therefore net transfer of volume from one system into the other, the output of one side will be falling, and that of the other will be rising. In addition, the volume changes in the two circuits will engender resistance changes. (If the volume of blood in one part of the circuit is raised, then the cross-sectional area of that part will increase, and the resistance across it will drop.) The resistance changes are in a direction which would tend to increase the inequality of stroke volumes, but this change will be compenstaed by adjustments of the stroke work equation which occur in response to a change in afterload.

2.23. Exercise

Under normal conditions the system operates in such a way that the volume shifts and pressure changes, which occur with changes in cardiac output, are small. Thus, with exercise, the large increase in cardiac output which occurs is obtained both by an increase in heart rate, and a very considerable shift upwards and to the left of the stroke work versus filling pressure equations, both wrought by sympathetic stimulation. Exercise is not associated with a rise in filling pressure unless the exercise is of very great severity or the heart abnormal.

Whatever changes are imposed upon the circulation—changes of posture, acceleration, exercise, haemorrhage, transfusion, vasoactive drugs—the components always adjust in such a way that the stroke volumes generated by the right and left heart become equal.

2.24. The model and its dangers

In the three foregoing sections of this chapter, a model of the central circulation has been constructed, and a theoretical background to the manner in which it might be disturbed in the face of ventricular dysfunction or alterations in the circulating volume has been established.

The model and the predictions about its distortion by disease led to the drawing of the three cartoons (Fig. 1) offered as a hypothesis in the first chapter, but physiological models are always dangerous. They blind their devotees to anything which is not compatible with the model.

The remainder of this book is offered as an answer to most reasonable distrust of the model. It is an account of the changes in stroke volume and stroke work of the two sides of the heart which accompany alterations in their filling pressures in a variety of clinical states.

2.25. Methods

In the ensuing studies, all pressures are related to zero at the sternal angle, and were measured with Statham P23Db transducers and recorded on an Ampex tape recorder. Mean pressures were obtained electronically. In cases subject to large intrathoracic pressure swings, the pressures recorded at end expiration have been used. In the case of patients being ventilated with intermittent positive pressure, all pressures were recorded at the end of expiration. Cardiac output was measured by a thermal dilution technique;[12] each point on the equations is the mean of five measurements of cardiac output divided by the heart rate at each determination.

Systemic arterial pressure was recorded through a short cannula in the femoral artery. Right atrial pressure was measured through a 20 cm catheter in the right internal jugular vein, advanced to the junction of the superior vena cava and right atrium. This catheter was also used for the injection of the thermal indicator (10 ml 5% dextrose at room temperature).

Filling pressure of the left heart was measured in most cases by retrograde catheterization of the left ventricle with a radio-opaque Teflon catheter (1 mm outside diameter). The approach was by Seldinger's technique from the femoral artery, and the filling pressure was measured as the end diastolic pressure in the left ventricle. In four cases left atrial pressure was measured by a modified trans-septal technique,[13] and in the case of acute nephritis, mean left atrial pressure was derived from the pulmonary arterial end diastolic pressure.[14] In the post-cardiac surgical cases, a Teflon catheter (0·4 mm internal diameter) was placed in the left atrium at the time of operation.

The pulmonary artery pressure was measured through a small nylon catheter (0·5 mm internal diameter) carrying a thermistor at its tip, which was used for measurement of the thermal dilution signal.

The atrial pressures were varied by the rapid removal of blood from the femoral vein through a short nylon cannula (1·4 mm internal diameter), using a 50 ml syringe. The blood was stored in ACD donor packs under sterile conditions. The volume removed between sets of flow and pressure measurements varied according to the compliance of the venous capacity bed, but was adjusted to create a suitable fall in atrial pressures.

Following the removal of each aliquot of blood, sufficient time was allowed for the pressures to become stable, and the pressure and flow measurements were then made.

3

The Overexpanded Circulation

3.1. The overexpanded circulation with a normal heart

Two examples in whom the relevant variables were determined will be discussed; both have the pattern of dysfunction that was proposed in the first cartoon (Fig. 1a), and although both were thought, on clinical grounds, to have heart failure, they were eventually shown to be suffering from an overexpanded circulating volume. The first was a 30-year-old diabetic man who had been found unconscious and hyperglycaemic, who had been treated with insulin and fluid replacement of an uncertain volume, but in excess of 4 litres, and who, in retrospect, was probably not dehydrated initially. On clinical examination the pulse rate was 90 in sinus rhythm, the jugular venous pressure was 10 cm above the sternal angle. Loud third and fourth heart sounds were audible over both ventricles. Blood pressure was 140/60. Respiratory rate was 30/min and diffuse crepitations were heard over both lung fields, and the liver was palpable. The patient was unconscious, both pupils reacted normally and doll's head eye movements were present. The corneal reflexes were present. The jaw jerk was pathologically brisk. Swallowing, pharyngeal control and the respiratory pattern appeared normal, apart from tachypnoea. The reflexes in the arms were abnormally brisk and the response to a painful stimulus was flexor (decorticate response). The reflexes and tone in the legs were normal, but both plantar responses were extensor. The urine contained sugar but no ketones. The blood sugar was 14 mmol/l (245 mg/100 ml). Chest x-ray showed mild pulmonary oedema and the heart size was within normal limits. The ECG was normal. The albumin level was 26 g/l, a matter of considerable importance, and the haematocrit 0·26. The albumin had been 35 g/l and the haematocrit 0·47 prior to the overgenerous fluid replacement.

Initially it was not realized that the circulatory abnormality was due to overexpansion of the circulating volume, and a diagnosis of heart failure and bilateral cerebral hemisphere lesions with an intact brain stem was made.

Investigation suggested that the patient had a normal heart, with both left and right ventricles producing high values of stroke work in response to high filling pressures. The equations of stroke volume in relation to filling pressure for the left and right heart are shown in Fig. 17.

It is the author's contention that these equations and the equations of stroke work related to filling pressure in Fig. 18, determined in this patient, represent the response of a normal heart to changes in filling pressure. The evidence for this proposition is:

(a) That the observed equations are straight line functions passing through normal values of stroke work and filling pressure, and stroke volume and filling pressure for both sides of the heart. (Left-sided filling pressure of +5 mm Hg corresponds to 68 gram metres, and right-sided filling pressure of −2 mm Hg to 12 gram metres.)

(b) That the stroke work equations correspond closely to the general equations developed from the information in Fig. 30. The general equation for left-sided stroke work

$$W_L = \frac{(b - 13)\,P_L + 10b - 130}{a + 10} + 13$$

produces a predicted equation

$$W_L = 3{\cdot}7\,P_L + 50$$

when a is +5 mm Hg and b is 68 gram metres, whereas the measured values give

$$W_L = 3{\cdot}1\,P_L + 53$$

If all the lower values of these equations represent the response of a normal heart to changes in filling pressure, there is no obvious reason for believing the heart to be failing at the higher values of filling pressure, in spite of the appearance of third and fourth heart sounds in the presence of the abnormally high filling pressures.

As will be seen, when the mean right atrial pressure is 4·4 mm/Hg, the stroke volume pumped by both right and left heart is 130 ml/beat and the left ventricular end diastolic pressure (LVEPD) 17·4 mm Hg.

A pulmonary capillary pressure of 17 mm Hg would not produce pulmonary oedema in the presence of a normal serum albumin level, but an albumin level of 26 g/l is probably associated with a critical value of pulmonary capillary pressure in the region of 15 mm Hg. This is in good accord with the values observed to be generating pulmonary oedema in this patient.

Once the diagnosis of overtransfusion was appreciated, the patient

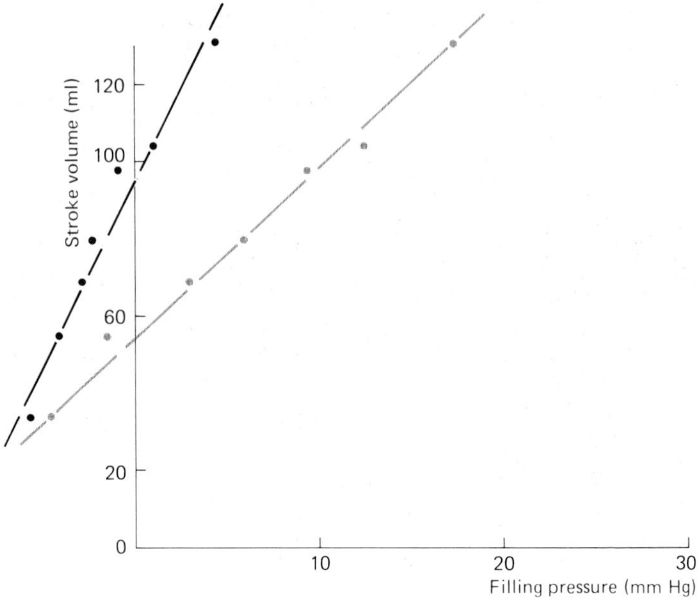

Fig. 17 Equations of stroke volume in relation to filling pressure for the left and right heart of a patient with a normal heart.

was treated by venesection. The volume which was removed in order to render the pressures and flows near normal (RAP −2·8 mm Hg, LVEDP 3·0 mm Hg, and a stroke volume of 69 ml/beat) was 2 litres. A further 1·5 litres was removed, bringing the pressures to much lower values (RAP −5·5 mm Hg, LVEDP −4·5 mm Hg) for a brief period of time, thus accelerating the reabsorption of the pulmonary oedema, with flows which remained adequate (cardiac output 4·2 l/min). The blood was then retransfused so that the right atrial pressure was held between −3 and −2 mm Hg, thus maintaining the left-sided filling pressure between +3 and +5 mm Hg, whilst a diuresis was provoked with frusemide. After eight hours all the blood which had been removed to gain rapid control of the situation, had been restored, without the prescribed limits set upon the atrial pressures being transgressed. The patient's circulation then behaved normally and continued to do so. The cerebral lesion showed gradual recovery with return to consciousness.

In the commentary on the cartoons, it was suggested that the failure of response of the overtransfused patient to treatment appropriate to heart failure, was due to the near parallel slope of the equations for the two sides of the heart. This prediction is only part of the explanation. The other part depends upon the very different state of the systemic venous capacity bed, which is dilated and full in overtransfusion, but less compliant (the venous tone is higher) in left heart failure.

The control of the pulmonary oedema in both this patient and a patient with severe heart failure (see section 4·6) requires that their left atrial pressures be reduced by a minimum of 10 mm Hg. In the overtransfused patient this required the removal of 1820 ml blood, as compared with only 340 ml for the same reduction in the patient with left heart failure; a ratio of 5·4 : 1. It is this very large discrepancy in the volume which must be removed to achieve control, which renders venodilators and diuretics relatively ineffective in the presence of potentially lethal overtransfusion.

The venous tone of the patient with heart failure is three times that of the overtransfused patient, if the venous tone is viewed as the reciprocal of compliance.

The compliance of the overtransfused patient's venous capacity bed* is 330 ml/mm Hg, and that of the patient described in section 2.4 with left heart failure due to acute myocardial infarction 90 ml/mm Hg; a ratio of 3·7 : 1. The two patients show a difference in sensitivity of the left atrial pressure to the removal of volume. Of this difference 60% is accounted for by the contrasting state of the venous tone, and 40% by the equations of performance of the two sides of the heart being more nearly parallel in the normal.

* This figure is not correct in absolute terms, but may legitimately be used for purposes of comparison. Colloid solutions which are added to the circulation are not necessarily distributed solely within the circulating space. However, all the performance equations detailed in this book were inscribed by moving from the highest filling pressures to the lowest by the rapid removal of blood, and so errors due to movement between the extracellular space and the circulating space are minimized.

An equally serious source of error stems from the fact that not all of the blood removed comes from the systemic venous capacity bed. The ratio of size of the systemic venous capacity bed and right heart in diastole on the one hand, to the pulmonary capacity bed and left heart in diastole on the other, is approximately 7 : 1. This, together with the fact that the pulmonary left heart system is less compliant, means that volume either added to or taken away from the circulation is likely to be distributed approximately 90% in the systemic circulation and 10% in the pulmonary. These values are approximations, but whatever the real ratio between the circuits, it is unlikely to change by a large measure. It is therefore legitimate to divide the gross volume change by the change in right atrial pressure which it produced, and to use the resulting figure of compliance of the systemic venous capacity bed for comparative purposes only.

3.2. Is there any clinical means of knowing that such patients are suffering from overtransfusion rather than heart failure?

Overtransfusion and heart failure are both accompanied by elevation of the atrial pressures, and the consequences of these—stiff lungs and pulmonary oedema. Both are likely to have third and fourth heart sounds over left and right ventricles. The outstanding differences between the two states are, in terms of cardiac output, venous tone and vascular resistance, and these provide the clinical physical signs upon which the diagnosis can usually be made.

The cardiac output in left heart failure may be normal or low, but it is never twice the normal resting value. In the overtransfused patient just described, the cardiac output was 11·9 l/min, the systemic vascular resistance one-third of normal (6·1 units instead of a normal 18 units), and a venous tone, as we have already seen, one-third of that in the patient with left heart failure. This combination of physiological changes produces abnormally warm, pulsating extremities and dilated peripheral veins, with a normal or mildly raised blood pressure.

3.3. The intercept on the abscissa

Before leaving the equations of stroke volume against filling pressure found in a normal heart, it is of interest that, were the equation for the right heart to be extrapolated to the left, it would cut the abscissa at a right atrial pressure of −10 mm Hg. This equates with the lowest values of right atrial pressure seen in patients with severe hypovolaemia.

3.4. The relation of stroke work and filling pressure in the normal heart

The stroke work of the left and right heart in relation to filling pressure is shown in Fig. 18. These equations and their slopes do not have quite the same significance as the equations determined by Sarnoff, Mitchell and Berglund in dogs, in which the afterload (that is, the resistance into which the ventricles were emptying) was maintained constant. At the upper end of each equation both the systemic and the pulmonary circulation were considerably overexpanded, and therefore their resistances abnormally low (SVR 6 units, PVR 0·25 units). At the lower ends of the equations, both circuits were mildly underfilled, and their resistances on the high side of normal (SVR 21 units, PVR 1·8 units). These complex changes which take place during the inscription of the 'work' curves detract from their value in terms of pure physiology (they are not

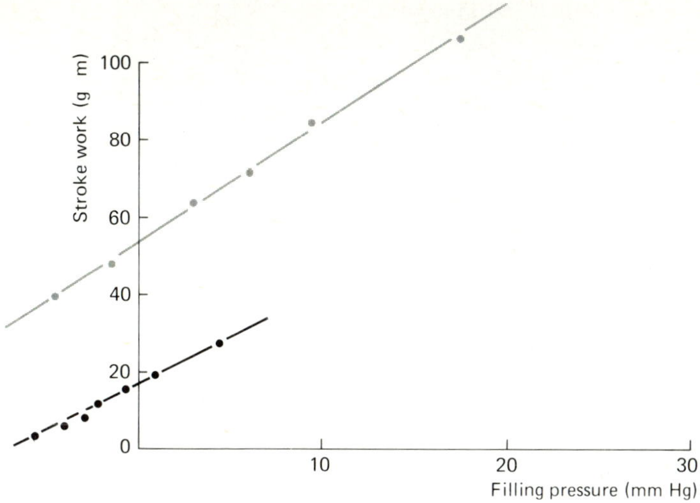

Fig. 18 Equations of stroke work of the left and right heart in relation to filling pressure of a patient with a normal heart.

strictly ventricular function curves because of the alteration in afterload), but for clinical management the information of greatest value is the behaviour of the entire reactive system as the filling pressures are manipulated.

3.5. Overexpansion of the circulating volume due to renal failure[15]

The second example of circulatory overexpansion occurred in a previously healthy 20-year-old man who was admitted with acute glomerulonephritis, subsequently confirmed histologically. On admission he was febrile (38°C) and dyspnoeic and had sacral and ankle oedema. Heart rate and blood pressure were both elevated (120/min and 170/100 mm Hg). The jugular venous pressure was 6 cm above the sternal angle, there were third heart sounds over both ventricles, and crepitations over both lung fields. The ECG was normal, and the chest x-ray (Fig. 19) showed bilateral pulmonary oedema. Urinary output increased within 48 hours of admission, but his dyspnoea worsened, and a diagnosis of polyarteritis nodosa with cardiac involvement was considered.

The equations of stroke volume in relation to filling pressure for both sides of the heart are shown in Fig. 20. The presenting values were a right atrial pressure of 5·3 mm Hg, a stroke volume from right and left heart of 111 ml and a left-sided filling pressure of 23·4 mm Hg.

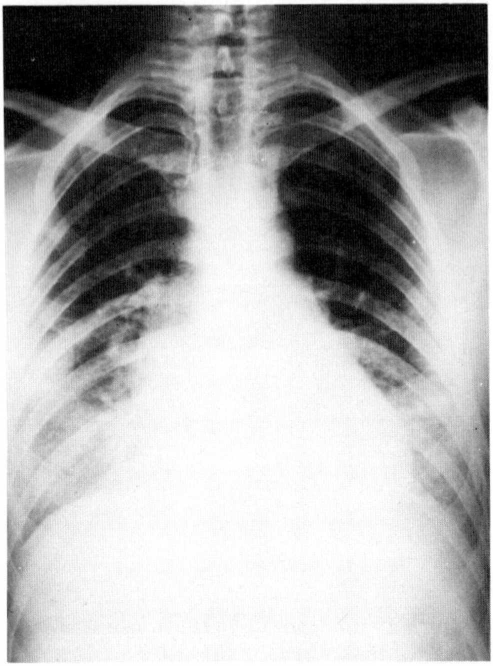

(a)

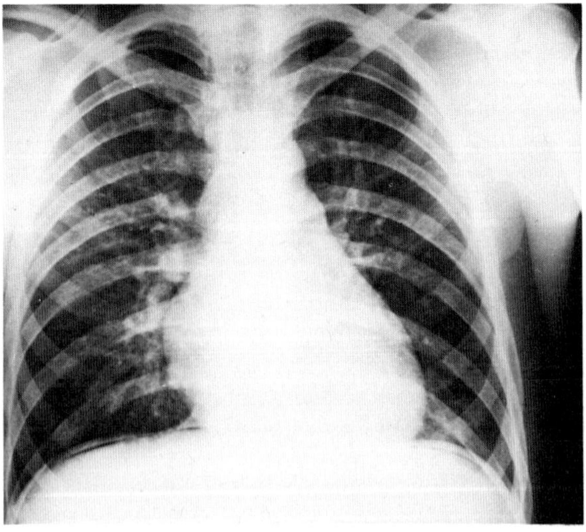

(b)

Fig. 19 Chest x-rays of a patient with acute glomerulonephritis (a) before, and (b) six hours after control of the pulmonary oedema by removal of circulating volume.

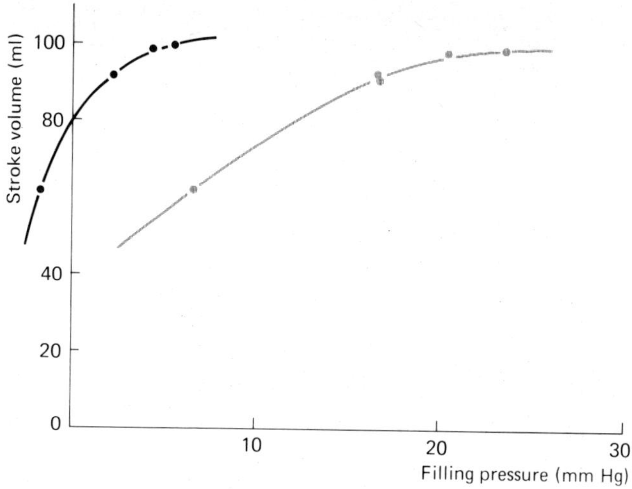

Fig. 20 Equations of stroke volume in relation to filling pressure for both sides of the heart of a patient with acute glomerulonephritis.

As in the previous patient, investigations suggested that the heart was probably normal, but operating with considerably raised atrial pressures, to produce a cardiac output of 11·9 l/min.

Retention of salt and water in acute nephritis dilutes not only the haemoglobin but also the serum albumin, and the albumin level of 28 g/l in this patient suggest that pulmonary oedema would be formed at pulmonary capillary pressures in excess of 16 mm Hg.

Reduction of the right and left atrial pressures and the stroke volume of the heart to normal values again requires the removal of a very considerable volume of blood (1400 ml), and again the compliance of the venous system is high (203 ml/mm Hg); that is, the venous tone is low. Also the systemic vascular resistance is very considerably reduced (8·5 units in relation to a normal of 18 units). The pattern of abnormality is similar to that demonstrated in the overtransfused patient, and the therapeutic implications are similar.

Haemodialysis is probably the ideal method of controlling all the abnormalities presented by this patient, both the hypervolaemia and the chemical consequences of his renal failure. If peritoneal dialysis is employed, as it was in this case, the initial effect of filling the abdomen with dialysis fluid would be to compress the venous capacity bed, and so raise the right atrial and therefore the left atrial pressure. This would increase the rate of formation of pulmonary oedema, and is thus potentially lethal. These hazards were avoided by removing a sufficient volume of blood to control the filling pressures before the institution of dialysis. The blood was preserved and retransfused after a sufficient volume of fluid had been removed by the dialysis.

3.6. Summary of the findings in the overexpanded circulation

(1) In spite of the clinical physical signs—a high venous pressure, abnormal heart sounds and pulmonary oedema—the patient may not be suffering from heart failure; both sides of the heart are producing a greater than normal stroke work, and when the filling pressures are reduced to normal the stroke work is normal. If the pulmonary oedema is sufficient to cause death then clearly the equations of function descend and ultimately coincide with the abscissa, but in the two patients described in this chapter, with moderate pulmonary oedema, the slope and intercept of the equations of function were demonstrated to be compatible with those of a normal heart.

(2) If the overexpansion of the circulation is life threatening, the most effective treatment is the removal of the excessive volume. This volume will be of the order of 1·5 litres.

(3) Therapeutic measures which are effective in left ventricular failure do not control the pulmonary oedema generated by volume overload in the presence of a normal heart. This failure is due in part to the low venous tone which implies very large volume changes to produce unit change in right atrial pressure, and in part to the near parallel condition of the equations of stroke volume for the right and left heart. This relation of the two sides of the heart means that an effective fall in left atrial pressure can only be achieved by a correspondingly large fall in right atrial pressure.

(4) The threshold pulmonary capillary pressure at which pulmonary oedema is formed in overexpansion of the circulation may be less than normal, because the albumin level is likely to be reduced.

4

Heart Failure

4.1. Definitions

Heart failure is here defined as an abnormality of the heart which interferes with its activity as a pump. This can be restated in terms of the physiology set out in Chapter 2, as an abnormality of the heart which interferes with its capacity to generate useful external work appropriate to the filling pressure. The simple version includes a judgement that it is the heart which is faulty. This separates abnormalities of the circulation, such as overexpansion and pulmonary embolism.

It is unreasonable to expect the division between normality and heart failure to be discreet, like a jump from one energy level to another; there are all shades of performance from normality to degrees of function insufficient to maintain life. The definition should not therefore be expected to provide a sharp separation between normality and failure.

The dissociation of the definition from physical signs similarly does no harm. It has been stated that 'the invariable characteristic of heart failure is congestion, and in the absence of congestion, there is no heart failure'.[16] This pattern of thought has led to a great deal of confusion. As has been pointed out at some length in Chapter 3, congestion does not always betoken heart failure. In this chapter it will become clear that the absence of congestion by no means excludes heart failure.

Poisoning of the renal tubules with diuretics is thought to improve the function of the ventricles as pumps, by reducing their contained volume and improving their efficiency in accord with Laplace's law. It may be that a heart so treated does become more efficient in terms of the relation between energy consumption and useful work generated, but inspection of the many equations relating stroke volume to filling pressure described in this book, reveals that an acute decrease in filling pressure is always accompanied by a decrease in stroke volume. It is of the utmost importance to realize that the patent's venous pressure may be reduced to normal and his pulmonary oedema cured by the exhibition of diuretics, whilst his heart remains grossly abnormal in terms of the stroke work and stroke volume generated in relation to filling pressure.

Indeed, were the clinician as aware of the cardiac output as he is of the pulse rate and blood pressure, he would know that in curing the pulmonary oedema with a diuretic, he had also reduced the cardiac output.

4.2. Poor flows and pulmonary oedema are separate syndromes

Heart failure may produce either pulmonary oedema or diminished flows or both, but it is vital to keep these two aspects of cardiac inadequacy entirely separate in any clinical assessment of a failing heart, even when they are both in evidence.

4.3. Analysis of a patient with both diminished flows and pulmonary oedema in terms of the model

The principles involved are best illustrated by factual examples.[13] A man aged 54, who was admitted to hospital following a second

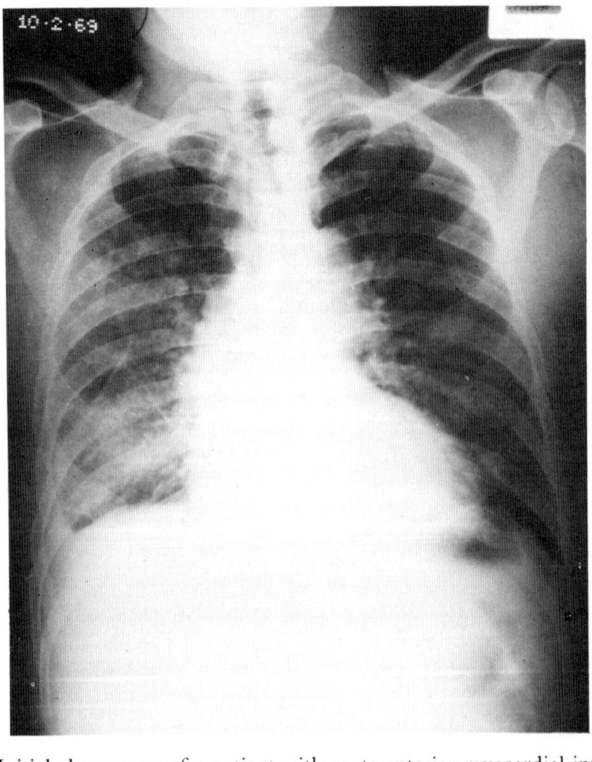

Fig. 21 Initial chest x-ray of a patient with acute anterior myocardial infarction.

episode of myocardial infarction, developed dyspnoea and orthopnoea early in the course of his illness. On examination he was in sinus rhythm with a heart rate of 112/min. The central venous pressure was raised 7 cm, and the heart moderately enlarged. Both third and fourth heart sounds were heard over both ventricles, but no murmurs were found. Blood pressure was 105/70. The extremities were cold and the peripheral veins constricted. Bilateral basal crepitations were heard and the chest x-ray (Fig. 21) showed some pulmonary oedema. The ECG showed evidence of a fresh extensive anterior myocardial infarct. In spite of treatment with digoxin, frusemide, ethacrynic acid, aminophylline and spironolactone, the patient's dyspnoea increased and after four days he had very severe pulmonary oedema (Fig. 22). Investigation at this time

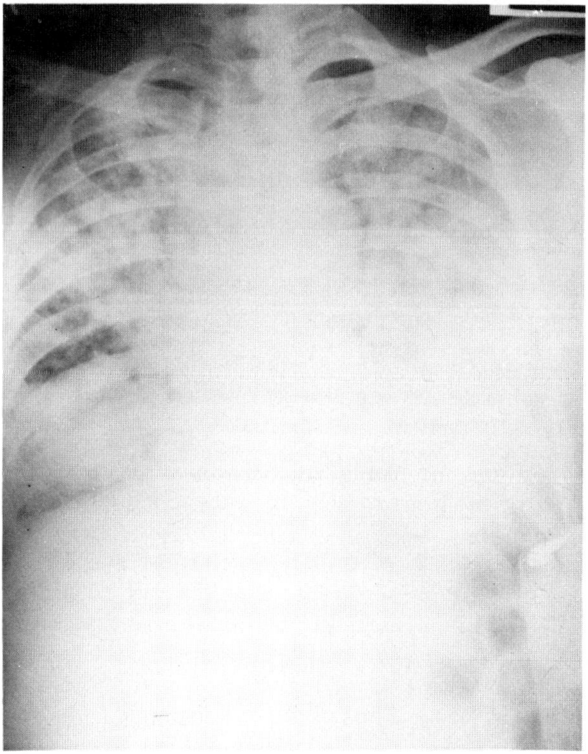

Fig. 22 Chest x-ray of the same patient as in Fig. 21, four days later, in spite of treatment with digoxin, frusemide, ethacrynic acid, spironolactone and aminophylline.

revealed a right atrial pressure of 7 mm Hg, a stroke volume of 27·6 ml from both sides of the heart and a left-sided filling pressure (LVEDP) of 30 mm Hg. This last figure, in conjunction with a serum albumin level of 42 g/l, accounts for the dense pulmonary oedema. A total of 420 ml of blood was removed from the circulation in three approximately equal venesections. Following the removal of each aliquot, observations of the pressures and flows were made. Figure 23 shows the relation of stroke volume to filling pressure for the left and right heart. It will be seen that, after the venesection,

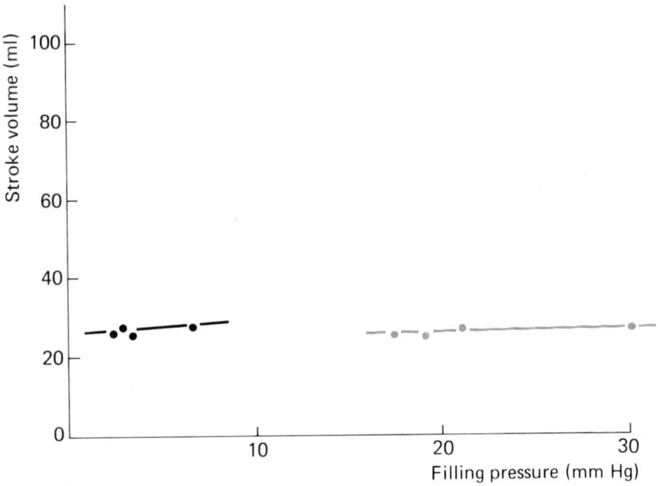

Fig. 23 The relation of stroke volume to filling pressure for the left and right heart of the patient with acute anterior myocardial infarction whose x-rays are shown in Figs. 21, 22 and 24.

the right atrial pressure had fallen to 2·3 mm Hg, the stroke volume of both sides of the heart to 26·5 ml and the left-sided filling pressure to 17 mm Hg.

Regulation of the left-sided filling pressure to this level was sufficient to control the pulmonary oedema, as will be seen from the chest x-ray (Fig. 24) taken ten hours later. These observations are in accord with the critical value of left atrial pressure for pulmonary oedema formation being in the region of 24 mm Hg for this patient (0·57 × albumin level). The fall in stroke volume from 27·6 to 26·5 ml was accompanied by a fall in pulse rate from 123 to 108/min; the cardiac output therefore fell from 3·4 to 2·9 l/min, thus control of the pulmonary oedema involved a further diminution of the already low cardiac output by 0·5 l/min.

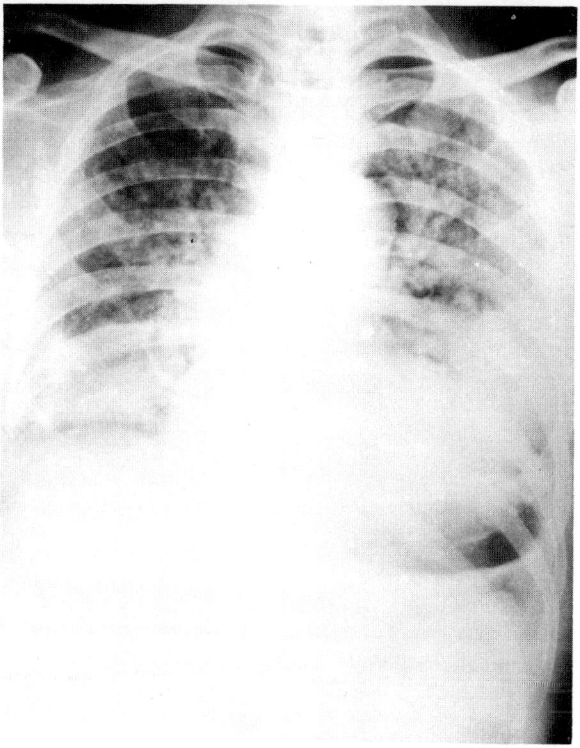

Fig. 24 Chest x-ray taken 10 hours after Fig. 22, showing partial clearing of the pulmonary oedema in response to control of the left atrial pressure.

4.4. The effect of isoprenaline

In the light of more recent experience, this patient would not be treated with inotropic agents, because the improvement in cardiac output which they produce can only be obtained by making the heart do more work. In the presence of a limited blood supply, which must be the case in ischaemic heart disease, this increase in work may well extend the area of the infarct, and certainly produces unwelcome biochemical changes.

At the time this patient was treated, it was thought that any improvement in cardiac output which could be obtained was beneficial and an intravenous infusion of isoprenaline was administered at a dose rate of 2 μg/min. The 420 ml of blood which had been removed was returned to the patient who then had a right atrial pressure of 0·8 mm Hg, a stroke volume of 49 ml from both right and left heart, and a left-sided filling pressure of 18·4 mm Hg. The change in the stroke volume relation with isoprenaline administration is shown in Fig. 25. The slopes for both right and left heart are considerably steeper, but the ratio of the slopes (left : right) of 3 : 1 remains unaltered, and the equations are still widely separated; fine control of the right atrial pressure is still important. A right atrial pressure of 0·7 mm Hg produces a stroke volume of 49 ml, and the left heart produces a matching stroke output when its filling pressure is 18·4 mm Hg, which is just within acceptable limits. (The

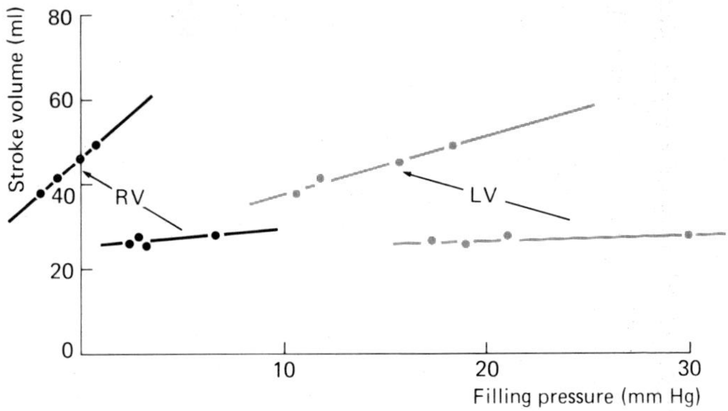

Fig. 25 The elevation of the stroke volume equations of the patient described in Fig. 23, with isoprenaline administration.

albumin level of 42 g/l implies a critical value of pulmonary capillary pressure in the region of 24 mm Hg.) Reduction of the right atrial pressure to −1·75 mm Hg reduces the stroke volume to 38 ml, which, at the heart rates involved, means a reduction in cardiac output of 1·5 l/min. Because of the relative slopes, it would only require a very small increase in the right atrial pressure to exceed the critical value for pulmonary oedema formation.

For the reasons detailed above, the patient's right atrial pressure was carefully controlled between zero and +1 mm Hg.

4.5. Isoprenaline and the venous capacity bed

Isoprenaline is normally a venoconstrictor, but in this patient it produces an increase in the compliance of the venous system from 93 ml volume change/mm Hg to 160 ml/mm Hg, a considerable fall in venous tone. As would be expected with this fall in venous tone, the right atrial pressure, with the same blood volume, falls (from 7 mm Hg to 0·7 mm Hg).

It is possible that this response of the venous system to isoprenaline occurs because it is being applied to a failing circulation, and the improvement in cardiac output induces the venodilatation.

4.6. Volume change and isoprenaline, and the systemic vascular resistance

As would be expected, the systemic vascular resistance falls as a result of isoprenaline administration. Also, as was demonstrated in the preceding chapter (section 3·4), the removal of blood from the system produces an increase in resistance across the vascular beds. In this case the 400 ml venesection produced a rise in systemic vascular resistance from 19·8 to 21·0 units in the absence of isoprenaline, and from 11·0 units to 14·5 during isoprenaline infusion.

4.7. The syndrome has been called left heart failure; is it really?

The syndrome which has just been examined in great detail is the clinical entity of left heart failure. When the equations of stroke work related to filling pressure of this patient are compared with those of the overtransfused patient with a normal heart (Fig. 26), it becomes obvious that right heart function is also impaired, and that in reality the patient has biventricular heart failure.

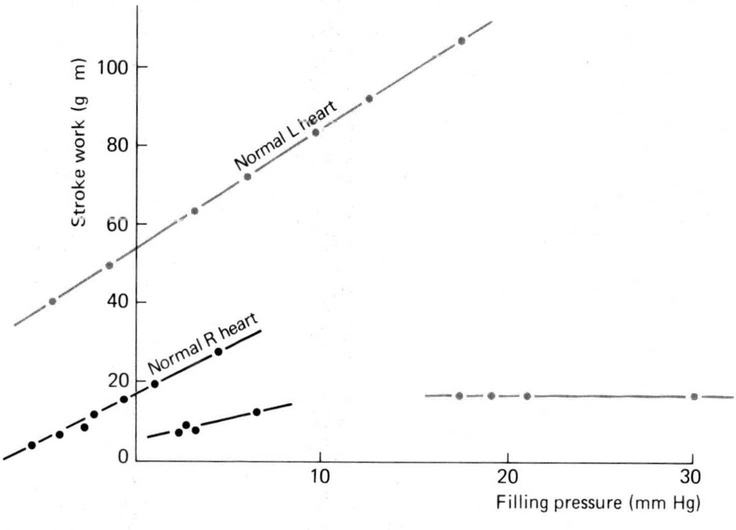

Fig. 26 Stroke work equations generated by the left and right heart of the patient with 'left' heart failure compared with those of a normal, showing that the right heart is also severely compromised.

4.8. The physiological characteristics of the left heart failure syndrome

The features of the disorder referred to as left heart failure which give it its clinical character (that is, liability to attacks of pulmonary oedema) are the ratio of the slopes of the stroke volume equations for left and right heart (Fig. 27), the wide separation of the equations and the relatively incompliant venous capacity bed. In this case

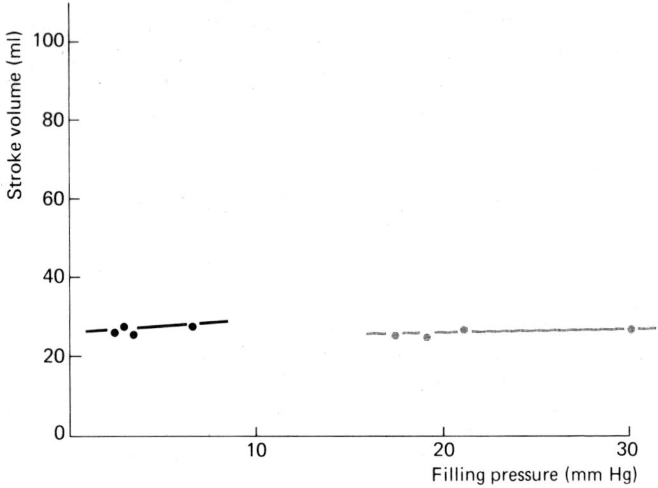

Fig. 27 In stroke volume equations associated with left heart failure, the equation of the left heart is shifted to the right, and is disproportionately flat when compared with the right heart.

the ratio of the slopes left : right is 3 : 1, implying that any change in right atrial pressure will be accompanied by an alteration in left atrial pressure three times as great; sometimes this ratio is considerably greater (Fig. 36).

The incompliant venous capacity bed, or high venous tone, in this instance is such that 93 ml of volume change produces a change in right atrial pressure of 1 mm Hg. These two features are additive and cause small changes in circulating volume to produce large changes in left atrial and pulmonary capillary pressure (34 ml volume change/mm Hg change in left atrial pressure in contrast to 182 ml/mm Hg in the overtransfused patient with a normal heart).

The same sensitivity of left atrial and pulmonary capillary pressure to small changes in volume, which makes the patient so prone to attacks of pulmonary oedema, also makes the condition readily amenable to treatment either by a small reduction in venous tone or circulating volume; a readiness, which as has been seen, is not shared by the overtransfused patient with a normal heart.

Patients with the 'left heart failure' configuration just described will, of course, become breathless at lower pressures than would occasion the generation of frank pulmonary oedema. As the point at which the patient is operating, on the equations of stroke volume versus filling pressure, moves to the right, there will be a net transfer of blood from the systemic into the pulmonary circulation, and with this increase in pulmonary blood volume the lungs will become stiffer.

4.9. Analysis of a patient with gross diminution of flows who is protected from pulmonary oedema

The second patient contrasts sharply with the one just described, although also suffering from myocardial infarction. He had collapsed suddenly and lost consciousness. With the return of consciousness, he complained of pain and tightness across the chest radiating to the left arm. Examination revealed restlessness, confusion, pallor, sweating, coldness of the extremities, a pulse rate of 84 suddenly falling to 44/min, jugular venous pressure +10 cm, blood pressure of 80/55 and the ECG changes of inferior myocardial infarction with complete heart block. The chest x-ray appeared normal.

A pacemaker was inserted via the right internal jugular vein, and ventricular pacing instituted. The heart rate was varied, and cardiac output was found to increase with heart rate from 1·1 l/min at 60 to 1·4 l/min at a rate of 100/min. Increase of rate beyond this failed to raise the cardiac output any further. The rate was therefore set at 100/min.

The extremely low values of cardiac output and the patient's condition suggested that every effort should be concentrated upon improving this value. An attempt was made to do this by raising the filling pressure with dextran. This is only admissible if the left-sided filling pressure is restricted to values below those at which pulmonary oedema might develop.

The relation of filling pressure and stroke volume for the right and left heart is shown in Fig. 28. The outstanding features are the close approximation of the equations and their extreme flatness. When the right atrial pressure was 7·4 mm Hg, the stroke volume of both sides was 13·5 ml, and the left-sided filling pressure (LVEDP) 7·4 mm Hg. When the right atrial pressure was 10·7 mm Hg, the left was 10·0, and the stroke output 14·0 ml. With a right atrial pressure of 22·0 mm Hg, the left was 14·2 and the stroke volume 15·0 ml.

The relation of performance of the two sides of the heart in this

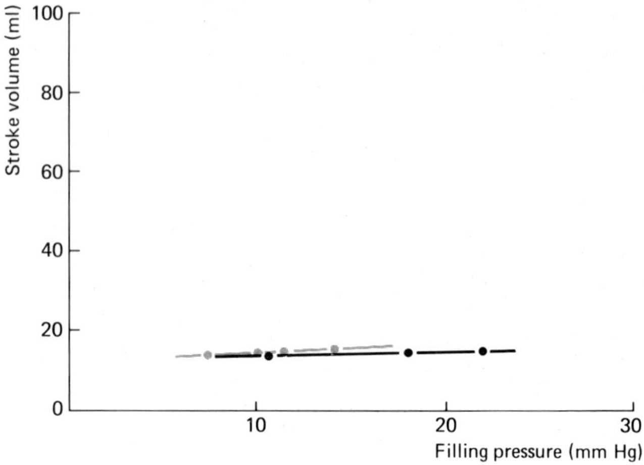

Fig. 28 Stroke volume equations of a patient with inferior myocardial infarction who has extreme impairment of stroke output, but is protected from pulmonary oedema by the transposition of the right heart equation to the right.

patient made the generation of pulmonary oedema impossible. However high the right atrial pressure, the left was always well below the level at which pulmonary oedema might appear. The outstanding problem remained the inadequacy of the cardiac output. (With the severely restricted cardiac output, the venous tone, when compared with the other patients so far discussed, was extremely high. The venous compliance calculated as stated in the footnote on p. 29 was 51 ml/mm Hg right atrial pressure change.)

4.10. Life-threatening impairment of cardiac output

It is a general truth, as was demonstrated in this patient, that if the cardiac output is impaired by heart failure to the point at which the lack of flows is life threatening, the equations of function will show extreme flattening. The implication of this flatness is that only trivial increases in cardiac output can be obtained by raising the filling pressure. In this case the cardiac output was 1·5 l/min when the right atrial pressure was 22 mm Hg, and 1·35 l/min with the right atrial pressure at 7·4 mm Hg. Under these conditions a useful increase in cardiac output can only be obtained by inotropic stimulation, which will move the whole equation upwards. In such grossly defective hearts, the response to an inotrope is also very limited. In this patient digitalization produced no measurable movement of the equations of stroke volume related to filling pressure. Isoprenaline administration (1·5 μg/min) improved the stroke volume equations by 2 ml/beat, raising the cardiac output to 1·7 l/min. So treated, the patient recovered.

4.11. The clinical and physiological characteristics related

Two contrasting examples of heart failure have been studied in some detail, and it has emerged that the nature of the clinical problem is related to five characteristics. These are:

(1) The flatness of the stroke volume equations, which, as they become flatter, reflect an increasingly inadequate cardiac output, and also make attempts to increase stroke volume by increasing filling pressure of less and less value.

(2) The relative slopes of the stroke volume equations for the right and left heart, which will determine the magnification factor between changes in right and left atrial pressure.

(3) The separation or approximation of the equations of stroke volume versus filling pressure for the right and left heart, which together with (2) will determine the minimum value of right atrial pressure at which the patient will generate pulmonary oedema.

(4) The state of the venous tone, which will enlarge or diminish the effect of a given change in circulating volume on the right atrial pressure.

(5) The serum albumin level, which, when multiplied by a constant (0·57), yields the approximate level of left atrial pressure at which the formation of pulmonary oedema will begin.

These factors will be examined in detail.

4.12. Depression of the stroke volume equations

In Fig. 29 the stroke volume equations of a normal left and right heart are compared with those observed in an extreme case of pump failure due to almost total infarction of the heart. The extent of the infarction was observed at post mortem. In Fig. 30 the stroke work equations of the same patients are compared. The patient with the myocardial infarct is a limiting case, the stroke volume equations being flat. In fact, each must have a very small positive slope, since a system with either flat or negatively sloping stroke volume curves would be unstable and the pulmonary circuit would either progressively fill or empty. Although the combination of a negatively sloping right-sided stroke volume equation and a positively sloping left is logically possible as a stable system, it is unlikely that it will ever be seen in nature because the right-sided stroke work equations, which have been observed, have a positive gradient until they coincide with the abscissa.

The negatively sloping equation of left-sided stroke work in

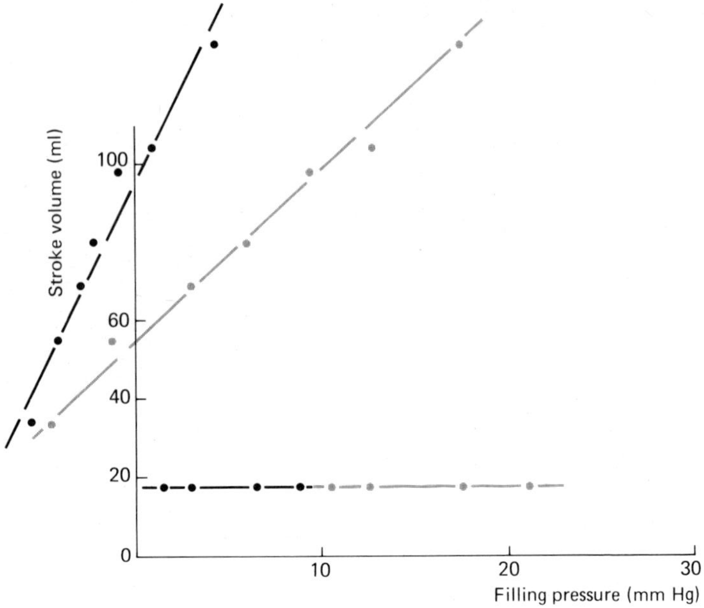

Fig. 29 Stroke volume equations of a case of extreme pump failure compared with those of a normal.

Fig. 30 correlates with the flat stroke volume equation in Fig. 29. Because, during the inscription of the equations, blood is removed from the circulation, there is a modest rise in the systemic vascular resistance; in this instance from 30·8 to 33·9 units. The increase in stroke work with diminishing left atrial pressure is balanced by the increasing systemic vascular resistance, and the net result is an unchanging stroke volume.

The equations of stroke work for the right and left hearts of a series of patients pumping from normal to the extremes of dysfunction are shown in Fig. 31. It is possible to develop general equations which approximate to these experimentally determined equations. The general equation for the left heart is

$$W_L = \frac{(b - 13)\,P_L + 10b - 130}{a + 10} + 13$$

where W_L is the stroke work of the left heart in gram metres, P_L is its filling pressure in mm Hg, and a and b are the x and y co-ordinates of any single point on the equation.

The fan-shaped arrangement of the equations implies that if the co-ordinates of a single point are known, the slope and intercept of

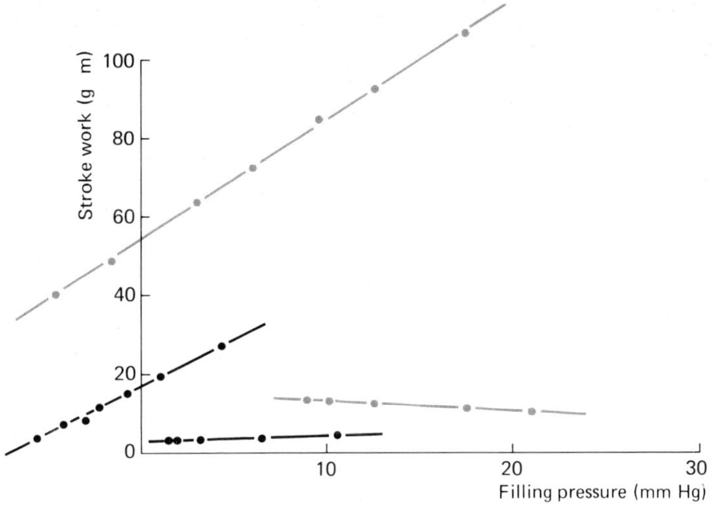

Fig. 30 Stroke work equations of the two patients illustrated in Fig. 29.

the equation passing through the point should be unique. The general equation for the right heart is

$$W_R = \frac{bP_R + 10b}{a + 10}$$

where W_R is the stroke work generated by the right heart in gram metres, P_R is its filling pressure in mm Hg related to the sternal angle, and a and b are the x and y co-ordinates of any single point on the equation. In this somewhat limited group all those patients whose left ventricular stroke work equations fell below 13 g m/beat in the absence of inotropic stimulation succumbed to inadequate flows. It is probably a mathematical accident that this is the level which coincides with the change from equations of positive to negative gradient.

At the lower end of the scale these equations of useful work generated in relation to filling pressure are a valuable quantification of heart failure. The capacity to generate an equation identical to that produced by a normal heart under these conditions does not unfortunately identify the heart as normal.

All the equations here described were obtained under 'resting' conditions, and a normal heart would undoubtedly develop much steeper equations under conditions of load, such as exercise. Minor degrees of 'failure' would only become apparent in these terms as an inability to meet the challenge of such a load. Moreover, the

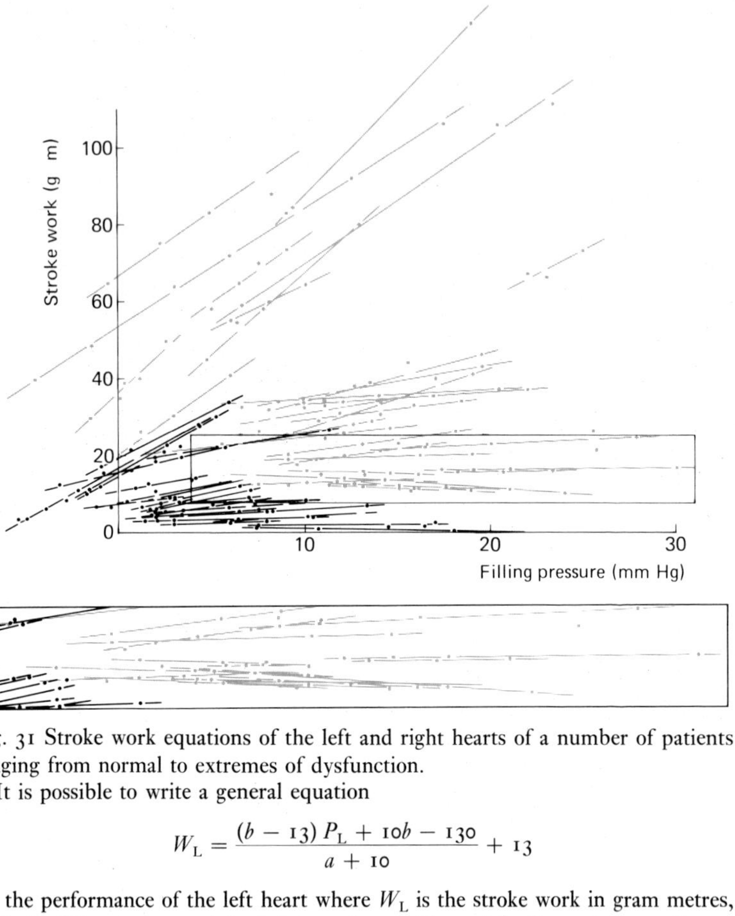

Fig. 31 Stroke work equations of the left and right hearts of a number of patients ranging from normal to extremes of dysfunction.

It is possible to write a general equation

$$W_L = \frac{(b - 13)\,P_L + 10b - 130}{a + 10} + 13$$

for the performance of the left heart where W_L is the stroke work in gram metres, P_L is the filling pressure of the left heart in mm Hg, and (a, b) are the co-ordinates of any one point on the equation. Thus if a point on the equation is known, a being the value of filling pressure and b the corresponding stroke work, substitution of the known values of a and b in the above equation gives an approximation to the equation which passes through the point. The general equation for the right heart is

$$W_R = \frac{bP_R + 10b}{a + 10}$$

where a is the known value of filling pressure and b the corresponding stroke work.

NB. If mid-chest were used as the manometer reference point in place of the sternal angle, the equations would become

$$W_L = \frac{(b - 13)\,P_L + 3b - 39}{a + 3} + 13 \quad \text{and} \quad W_R = \frac{bP_R + 3b}{a + 3}$$

Inset shows expanded version of outlined portion

quantification of heart failure in these terms makes no distinction between dysfunction due to defects of valve or muscle, and is inappropriate if these are the questions at issue.

4.13. The area of uncertainty

In the group suffering from acute myocardial infarction shown in Fig. 32, patients with levels of left ventricular performance down to equation A will survive without inotropic stimulation. Those with levels of function below equation B all died from inadequate flows

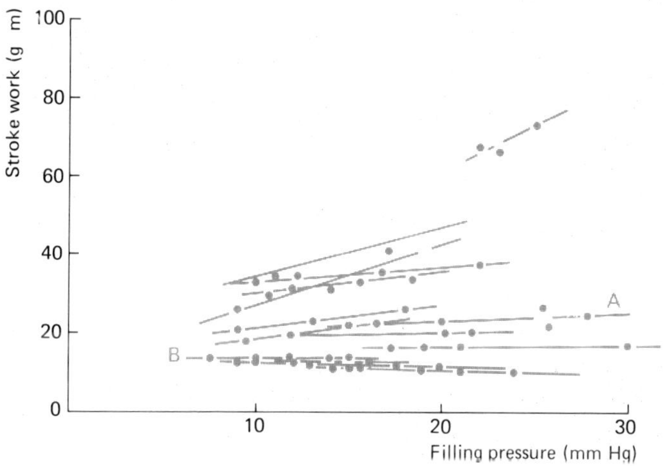

Fig. 32 The stroke work equations, without inotropic stimulation, of the left hearts of a group of patients suffering from acute myocardial infarction. Those above and including A, with a gradient greater than 0·3, all survived without inotropic stimulation. Those below B, with gradients less than 0, all died from inadequate flows however treated.

however treated, and, at post mortem, after periods of inotropic support from two to ten days, all showed massive infarction involving almost the entire heart.

There is an area of uncertainty between A and B, that is between the equations $W_L = 0{\cdot}29\ P_L + 16$ and $W_L = 0{\cdot}05\ P_L + 13{\cdot}5$. The very small number of patients in this series, whose left-sided function fell within this window, were treated with inotropic agents, and all have survived for relatively long periods of time. As already pointed out, the increase in work and myocardial oxygen consumption produced by the inotropic agents in the presence of a limited blood supply is likely to extend the area of infarction,[17] and has also been demonstrated to produce undesirable biochemical changes in the coronary circulation.[18] It is possible that these patients might ultimately have had better function had they not been stimulated with catecholamines, but it is also possible that they might have died of inadequate flows during the acute stage.

4.14. Severe flow failure

The point has already been made that if the degree of failure is life threatening, in terms of inadequacy of flows, the equations of stroke volume will have so little slope that attempts to improve the cardiac output by raising the atrial pressures will be of little value.

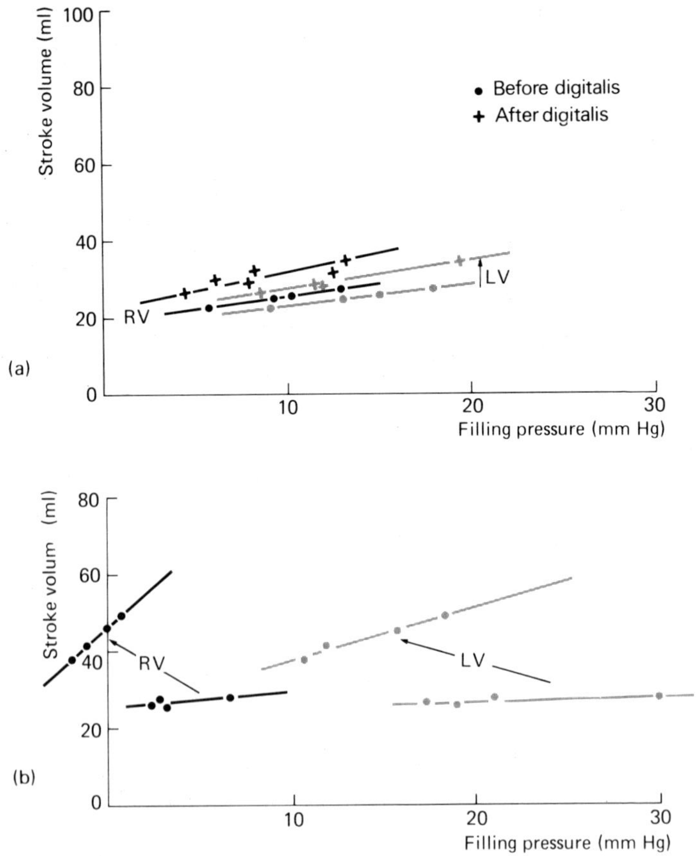

Fig. 33 (a) The effect of digitalization contrasted with (b) stimulation with isoprenaline in patients with acute myocardial infarction. Isoprenaline produces a greater shift of the equations upward and to the left.

Inotropic stimulation will improve the flows under these conditions, lifting the entire equation upwards; digitalis has less effect than isoprenaline, as is shown by the examples in Fig. 33. Also as might be expected, as the state of the heart deteriorates, the improvement which can be obtained with any inotropic stimulus diminishes. In the example shown in Fig. 34, digitalization had no effect on the equations, and isoprenaline produced only a very

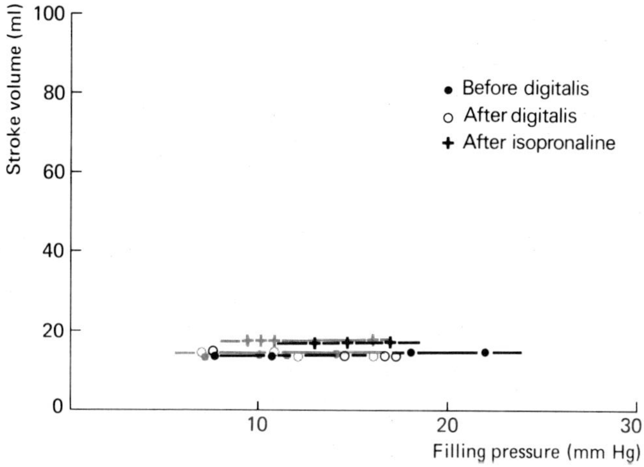

Fig. 34 With extreme impairment of function the stroke volume equations (●) are flat, so that stroke volume cannot be increased by adjustment of the filling pressures. Digitalization (○) produced no change, and isoprenaline (+) a very modest elevation of the equations.

modest increase in stroke volume. Under these conditions, in the absence of ischaemic heart disease, it would seem logical to use the most effective inotropic agent available.

4.15. Lesser degrees of flow failure

With intermediate degrees of failure, digitalis has the advantage that it can be taken by mouth, and it will be inotropically effective. Also the stroke volume equations have an appreciable positive gradient so that an increase in atrial pressures will raise the cardiac output. The limit upon this latter device for achieving better flows is simply breathlessness, this being the clinical indicator that the left atrial and pulmonary capillary pressures are rising to a level which is making the lungs stiff, if not flooding them with oedema.

Clinically this proposition should perhaps be made in reverse, and the plea made that, if the equations of stroke volume for the two sides of the heart are set close together and the atrial pressures

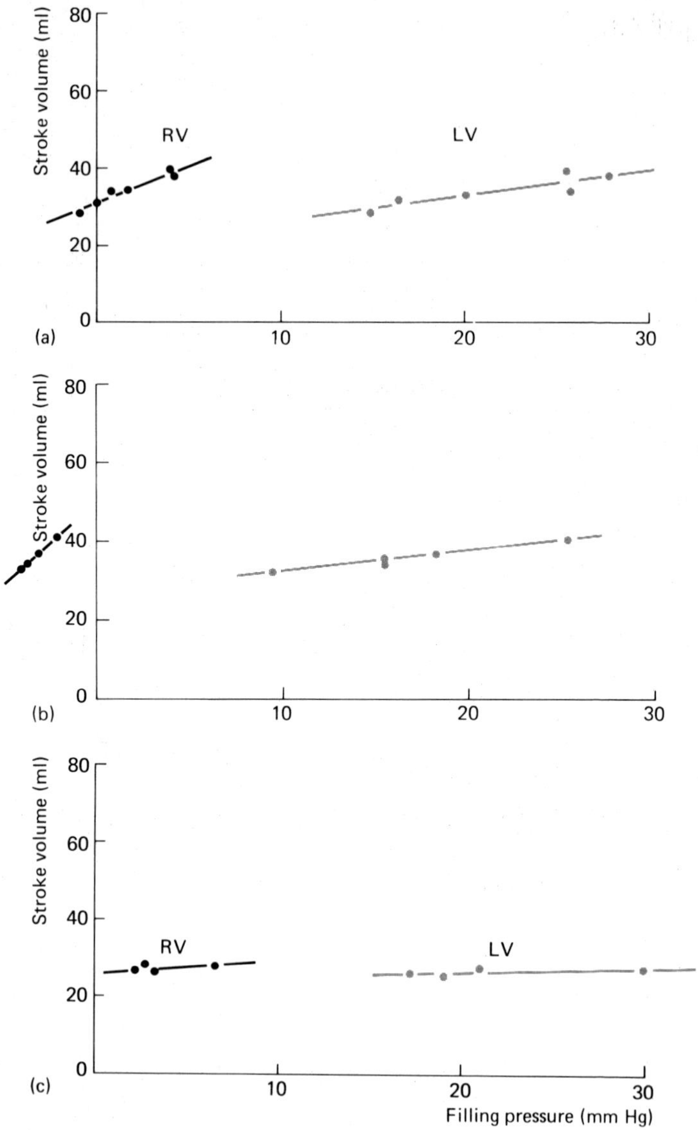

Fig. 35 (a), (b) and (c) Equations of stroke volume in acute anterior myocardial infarction showing wide separation of the equations and consequent susceptibility to pulmonary oedema.

(d) and (e) From cases of acute inferior infarction. The relation between left and right atrial pressures preserves the patient from pulmonary oedema, and reduction of the right atrial pressure will only diminish the stroke volume. (f) Inferior infarc-

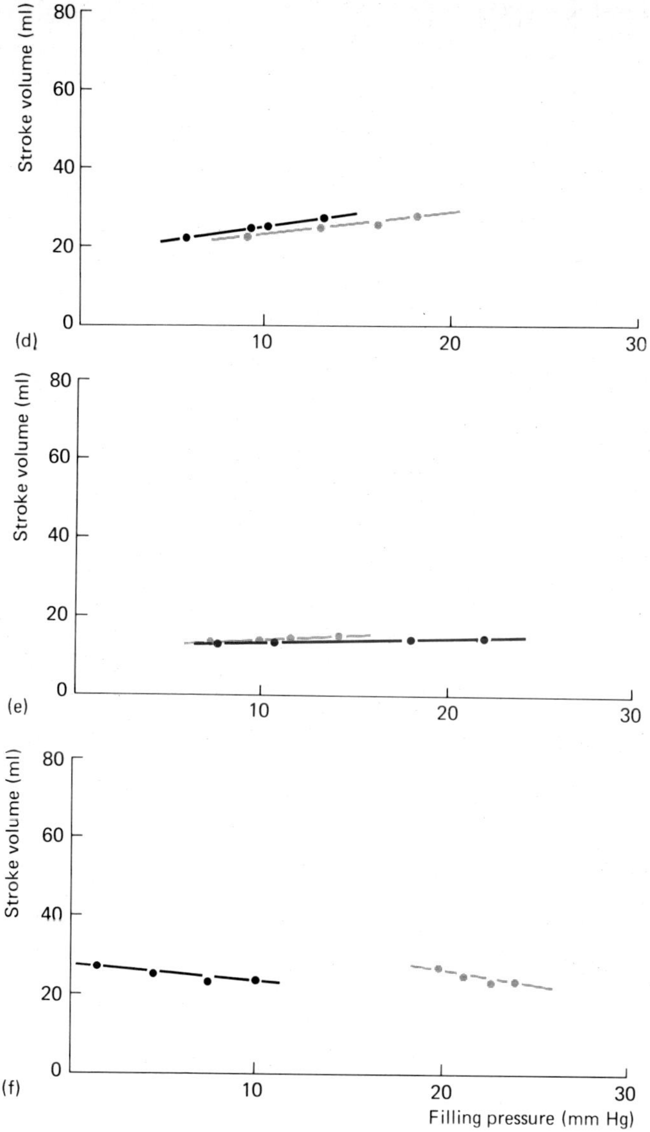

tion complicated by inferior papillary dysfunction, and mitral regurgitation producing separation of the equations similar to that seen in anterior infarction.

The theoretically impossible negative slope of the stroke volume equations is probably associated with an alteration in the contractile state, due to decreasing mitral regurgitation during the inscription of the equations, as a result of the removal of circulating volume.

therefore nearly identical, then it can only be detrimental to the patient to lower the right atrial pressure with diuretics. If the atrial pressures are widely separated then clearly diuretics are indicated.

How is the clinician without special measuring facilities to know that the equations of function are closely apposed? The absence of dyspnoea or pulmonary oedema in the presence of a high right atrial pressure suggests this pattern, and the absence of breathlessness on exertion makes the probability high. (Exercise raises the right atrial pressure in the presence of a failing circulation.)

4.16. Sites of infarction and patterns of dysfunction

In the presence of acute inferior (diaphragmatic) myocardial infarction, the stroke volume equations of the two sides of the heart are close together; in acute anterior infarction they are widely spaced. Examples are shown in Fig. 35. Clinically this means that in uncomplicated inferior infarction, an elevated right atrial pressure may, and often should, be left untreated,[19] whereas in acute anterior infarction, modest or even normal levels of right atrial pressure may be associated with an unacceptably high left atrial pressure, and demand the use of diuretics. Lateral extension of an inferior infarct produces an intermediate degree of separation of the equations. The complication of diaphragmatic infarction by inferior papillary muscle dysfunction, and acute mitral regurgitation, produces wide separation of the equations (Fig. 35f). Pre-existing old anterior infarction also causes separation of the equations.

4.17. The attempt to improve flows by removing the afterload

There is a possible solution to the dilemma which arises in the treatment of extremes of heart failure due to ischaemic disease, where the cardiac output is inadequate, and yet inotropic stimulation is only likely to extend the myocardial damage. It has been suggested that if the afterload upon a failing ventricle were removed, the same flows should be generated for less work, or that with the same work the flows might be better (see section 2.20).

A number of agents have been used for this purpose; most of them are α-blocking agents with a very short duration of activity. Given as a continuous intravenous infusion, they allow the arterial pressure to be lowered in a controlled fashion. Sodium nitroprusside and phentolamine have both been used. The effect of this manoeuvre upon the function of a patient with acute anterior myocardial infarction is shown in Fig. 36. The patient's pulmonary oedema is cured dramatically (Fig. 37), but there is no significant change in the slope of either the stroke volume or the stroke work equations following the nitroprusside infusion (100 mg/min). The dramatic improvement in the patient's pulmonary oedema has occurred because the systemic venous capacity bed has dilated so that, for the same contained circulating volume, the right atrial pressure has fallen. In

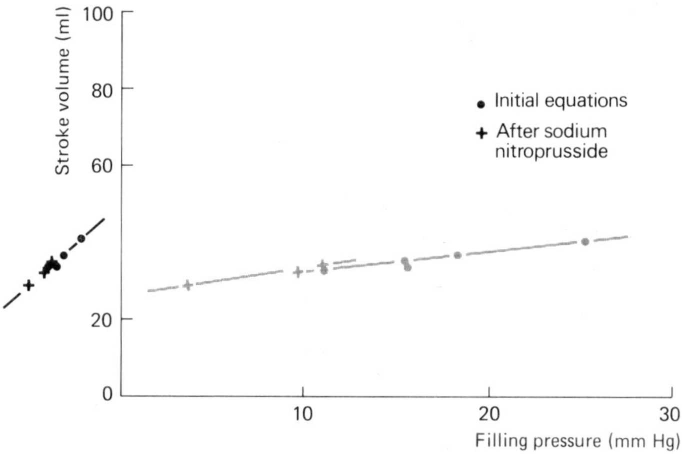

Fig. 36 The stroke volume equations of a patient with acute anterior myocardial infarction (●) are moved to the left (+) by sodium nitroprusside. The increase in slope of the left-sided equation is insignificant. There is an increase in cardiac output due to an increase in heart rate from 90 to 100/min.

this patient the ratio of slopes left : right is 7·5 : 1, and the separation of the stroke volume equations so extreme that the patient has a left-sided filling pressure of 25 mm Hg when the right is −2 mm Hg (serum albumin 36 g/l). The reason for the very wide separation is apparent in the stroke work equations (Fig. 38); that for the right heart is within normal limits, whereas the left is grossly impaired.

The magnitude of the movement of the function curves produced by Sarnoff by varying the afterload was small compared with that produced by inotropic stimulation in normal dog hearts.[11] It might be expected, therefore, that where the heart is so grossly disturbed that its response to inotropic stimulation is small, the changes produced by reduction in the afterload might be difficult to measure.

The outstanding characteristic of a severely failing heart is a fixed low stroke output, not easily altered by treatment.

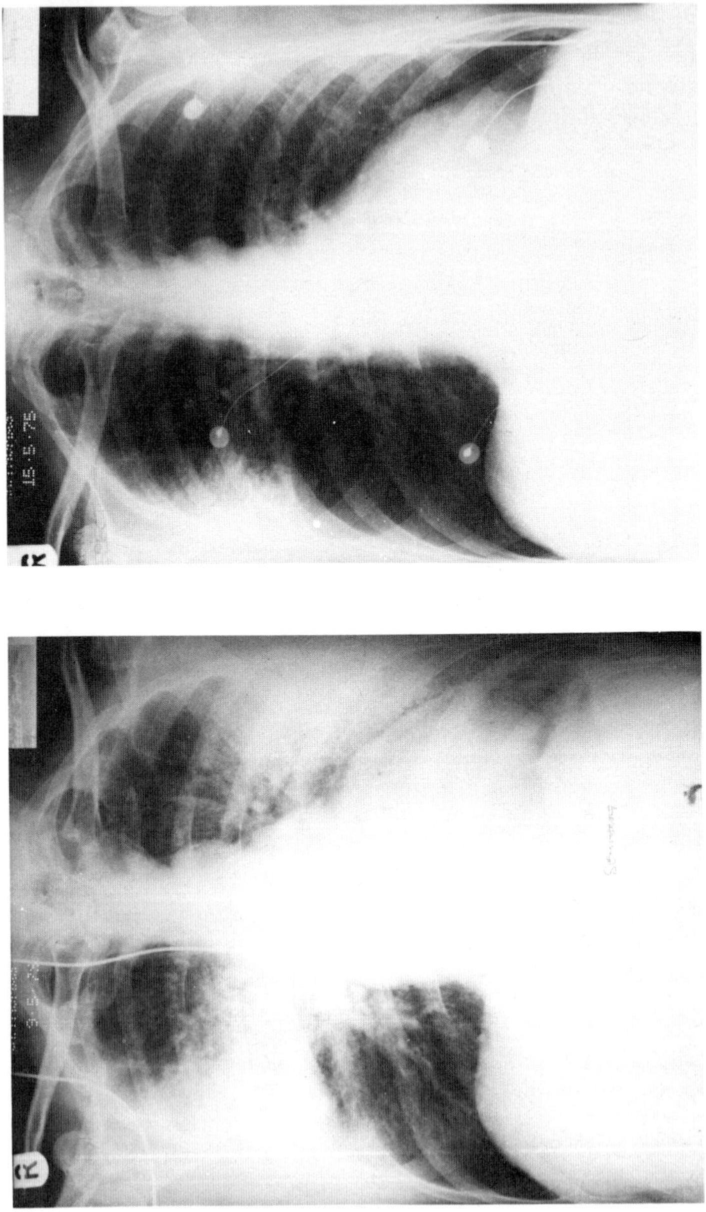

Fig. 37 Control of (a) pulmonary oedema following (b) the decrease in left atrial pressure produced by the sodium nitroprusside.

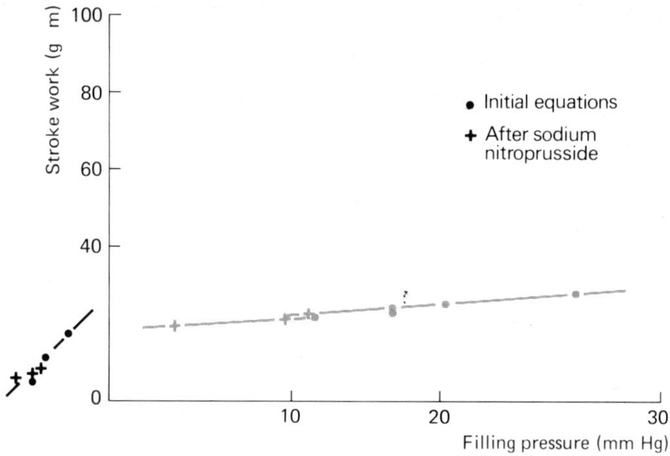

Fig. 38 The stroke work equations of the patient show the same movement to the left with sodium nitroprusside. The decrease in the slope of the left-sided equation is insignificant. The function of the right heart has been little impaired by the infarct.

4.18. Why should pulmonary oedema not be treated by the administration of albumin?

The critical value of pulmonary capillary and left atrial pressure at which pulmonary oedema develops is related to the level of circulating albumin as was shown by Guyton.[2] It would seem possible, therefore, that pulmonary oedema might be treated by raising the albumin level. Salt-free albumin given in normal concentration raises the right atrial pressure, and, if given in high concentration with the intention of avoiding the circulatory volume load, still produces a rise in right atrial pressure, by attracting fluid from the extracellular space. The possible benefits in the acute situation always appear to be offset by the attendant rise in atrial pressures.

5
A Raised Pulmonary Vascular Resistance

5.1. The third cartoon

The third cartoon (Fig. 1c) was said in the first chapter to have been drawn as a matter of logical necessity. It is always reassuring to discover that something which appears to be a logical necessity can exist outside the mind.

5.2. Movement of the stroke volume equations

There is a basic principle governing the movement of the stroke volume equations which has not yet been stated. These equations will be moved to the right, either by depression of the stroke work equation or by an increase in the resistance into which the ventricle is discharging its load, and moved to the left by an improvement in the stroke work equation or a decrease in the resistance. This means that the stroke volume equations will be moved farther apart from their normal positions either by depression of function of the left heart or by an increase in the systemic vascular resistance, and will be brought together by depression of function of the right heart or an increase in the pulmonary vascular resistance. These observations are supported by the work of Cohn.[20]

The principle has already been observed in the contrast between the findings in acute anterior and acute inferior myocardial infarction (section 4.16), where the observed changes were due to relatively greater depression of the right-sided stroke work in inferior infarction, and of the left in anterior infarction.

The validity of the principle in relation to changes in the systemic vascular resistance, might be thought to have been called in question by the finding that reduction of the left ventricular afterload with sodium nitroprusside (section 4.17) failed to produce a measurable alteration of the relation between the right and left atrial pressures. This apparent failure is almost certainly a question of degree, since the fall in systemic vascular resistance produced by reduction of the systolic blood pressure from 95 to 80 mm Hg with sodium nitroprusside was only from 22·3 to 19·8, an 11% change.

The increase in pulmonary vascular resistance which, as will be seen, produces a dramatic movement of the stroke volume equations is a change of 1400%, a change of a very different order.

A detailed clinical account of this patient is included as it may help to underline the consequences to such patients of treatment with diuretics.

5.3. Analysis of a patient with an acute pulmonary embolus

A woman of 66 years weighing 113 kg was admitted with a history of sudden onset of dyspnoea and central chest pain whilst climbing the stairs. The dyspnoea had increased in the 24-hour period between its onset and the patient's admission to hospital. The pain had been central substernal in distribution, radiating to the left shoulder, and had lasted between two and three hours. Examination revealed that the patient was extremely obese and dyspnoeic but not orthopnoeic. The pulse rate was 92 in sinus rhythm, and the venous pressure 7 cm above the sternal angle. The heart was enlarged, and third and fourth heart sounds were heard. Blood pressure was 110/70. The respiratory rate was 32/min and crepitations and expiratory ronchi were heard all over the chest. Observation of the state of the peripheral veins was impossible because of the obesity, but the extremities were reported as cool. The chest x-ray showed moderate cardiac enlargement, and the ECG inverted T waves in the lateral chest leads, but no other abnormality.

A diagnosis of heart failure due to ischaemic heart disease was made, and treatment with diuretics (frusemide) instituted. During the ensuing three days a moderate diuresis occurred, and the venous pressure was reported to have fallen toward, but not as far as, normal. The patient was alone in feeling that she had not improved. On the third day the patient was placed in a sitting position with her legs dependant. She became syncopal and developed extreme bradycardia. Cardiac massage was instituted, and the systolic arterial blood pressure returned to 90 mm Hg.

At this time the patient was transferred for investigation. The physical findings were as reported above. Again, adoption of the sitting position with the legs dependant produced syncope and intense bradycardia, which were treated with atropine and cardiac massage, and again the systolic blood pressure was restored to 90 mm Hg.

The combination of a raised venous pressure and postural hypotension on the one hand, and the suspicion that patients with extensive pulmonary embolism might behave in the manner of the third cartoon (Fig. 1c), suggested the diagnosis of pulmonary embolism.

Pulmonary angiography was performed using a portable image intensifier, and the images recorded on a video-recording system.

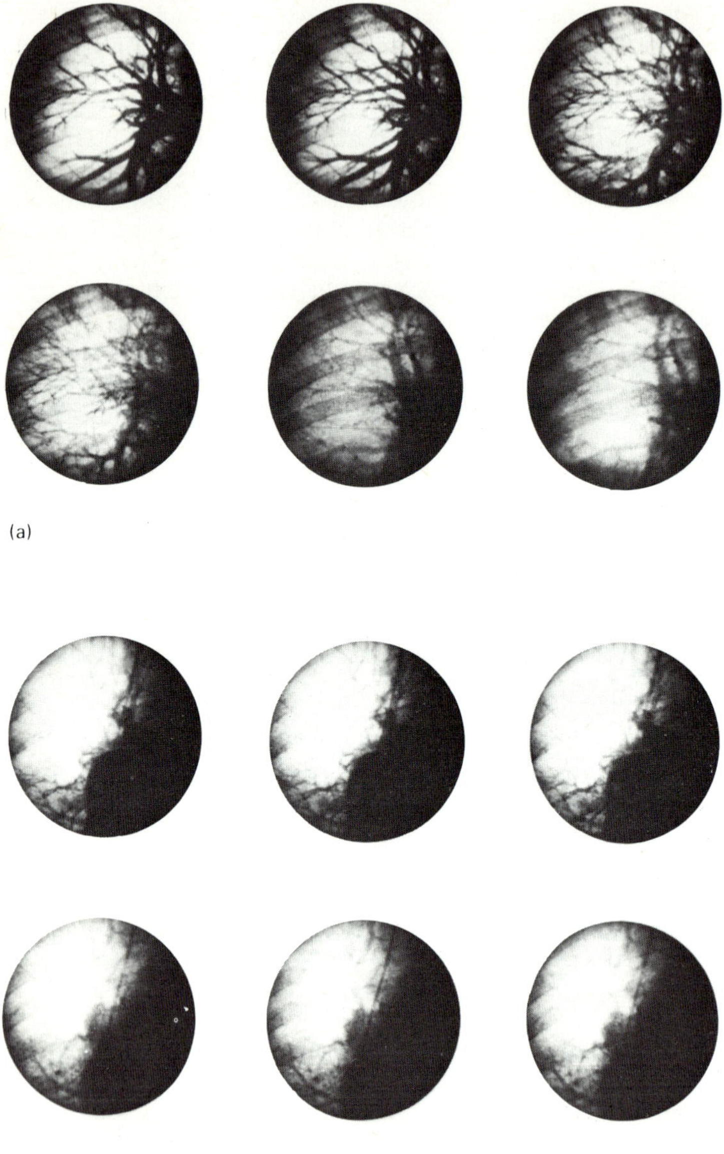

(a)

(b)

Fig. 39 Frames from bedside pulmonary angiograms using portable image intensifier (Siemens Siremobil 2) and video-recorder (International Video Recorders). (a) A near-normal right lung. (b) The right lung of the patient showing near-complete obstruction.

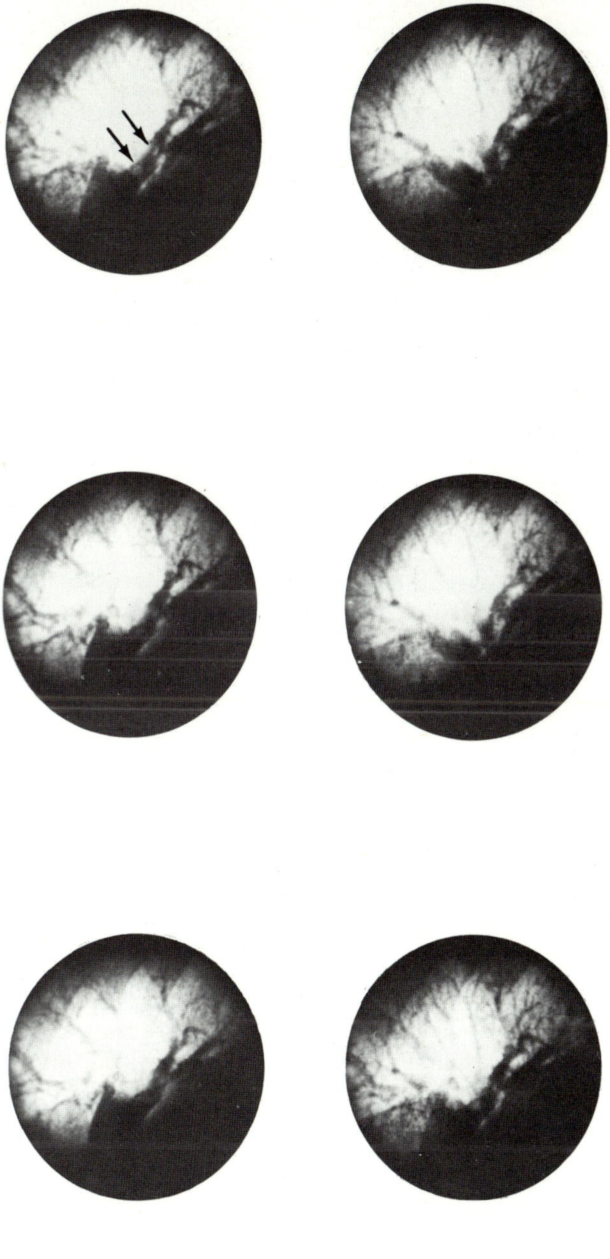

(c)

Fig. 39(c) Left lung of same patient showing considerable obstruction with pulmonary emboli (filling defects arrowed).

Figure 39 shows a number of frames recorded in this manner from a near normal right lung (a); (b) and (c) are similar frames from the patient, and show occlusion of major portions of both lungs with pulmonary emboli.

Treatment with the diuretic was stopped and heparinization commenced. A study was undertaken to ascertain the effects of raising the right atrial pressure, as the patient had twice demonstrated that lowering of the right-sided filling pressure was disastrous.

The results of the investigation are shown in Fig. 40; the stroke volume equations are arranged as they were in the third cartoon.

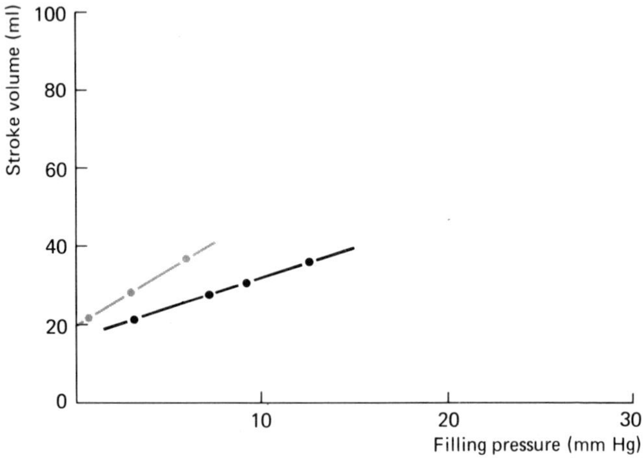

Fig. 40 The equations of stroke volume in acute pulmonary embolism are laterally transposed, as they were in the third cartoon (Fig. 1c).

The equation for the right heart is shifted so far to the right that it moves beyond that of the left heart, and they become laterally transposed. At the commencement of the study, with a right atrial pressure of 3 mm Hg, the stroke output of both sides of the heart is 21 ml, and the left-sided filling pressure (LVEDP) 0·7 mm Hg. After transfusion with 500 ml of Dextran 70 in 5% dextrose (an artificial plasma expander), the right atrial pressure had risen to 12·5 mm Hg, the stroke volume to 36 ml and the left-sided filling pressure to 6 mm Hg. The cardiac output had been raised from 1·9 to 3·1 l/min by raising the right-sided filling pressure to a level which would embarrass a normal heart. This without the left-sided filling pressure (LVEDP) rising beyond normal. The high resistance produced by the pulmonary emboli is at arterial and arteriolar level; the capillaries are distal to this resistance and in free communication with the left atrium. The pulmonary capillary pressure therefore was also normal, and the remaining functional part of the pulmonary vascular bed not liable to pulmonary oedema.

Pulmonary oedema has been reported in lungs affected by pulmonary emboli, and would be extremely likely to form in those parts of the vascular bed which had been subject to occlusion for a sufficient time for the capillary endothelium to be damaged. In the special case of the lung, the non-perfused endothelium should not suffer from gross hypoxia, but might well suffer from other biochemical changes due to lack of substrates.

The change in cardiac output from 1·9 to 3·1 l/min cannot be accounted for simply by the increase in stroke work generated by the right heart. The equations of stroke work against filling pressure for the left and right heart are shown in Fig. 41.

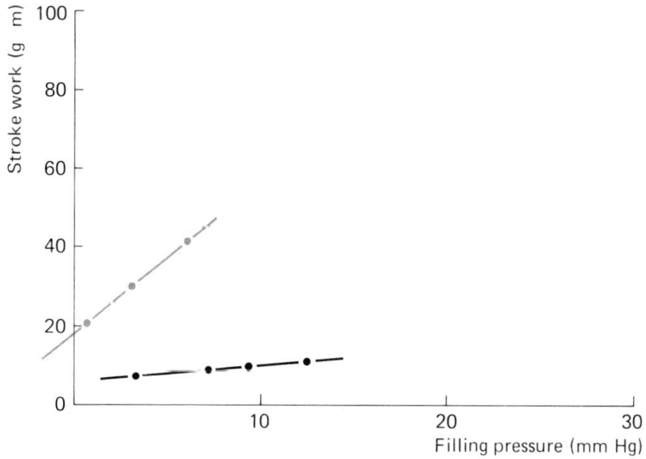

Fig. 41 The equations of stroke work in acute pulmonary embolism. The increase in the stroke work of the right heart, which occurs with elevation of the right atrial pressure, is insufficient to explain the increase in stroke volume seen in Fig. 40.

The stroke work of the right heart increased from 7 to 11 gram metres as the right atrial pressure was raised from 3 to 12·5 mm Hg. This increase in work produced by the right heart is insufficient to explain the rise in stroke volume from 21 to 36 ml. Another change has taken place at the same time: the pulmonary vascular resistance has fallen from 14 to 9 units. It is reasonable to suppose that some part of this fall in resistance of the pulmonary bed is due to the expansion of that bed by the Dextran. The major proportion of the Dextran will have been distributed into the systemic venous capacity bed, but a fraction of it must have been distributed into the pulmonary capacity bed because the LVEDP has risen from 0·7 to 6 mm Hg. (The fraction would be of the order of one-seventh if the compliance of the systemic venous capacity bed and right heart were the same as that of the pulmonary venous capacity bed and left heart, but because the latter is a stiffer, less compliant system, the fraction will be less.)

The change in pulmonary vascular resistance which occurs during the inscription of the equations has the effect of making the right-sided stroke volume equation steeper than it would otherwise be.

5.4. The consequences of the high pulmonary vascular resistance, lateral transposition pattern

The logical consequences of this arrangement of the equations in acute major pulmonary embolism have considerable bearing upon the management. The right atrial pressure should be kept high; on the evidence so far available, a positive value of 12 mm Hg above the sternal angle appears appropriate to provide optimal right-sided stroke work in acute major pulmonary embolism. The advantages of greater elevation of the right atrial pressure are vitiated by problems such as pain from stretching of the hepatic capsule, increasing tricuspid incompetence and overstretching of the right ventricle.

The remaining pulmonary vascular bed should be kept well filled to keep its resistance value down. This is implicit in maintaining a high right atrial pressure. Dextran is a suitable fluid because the venous tone is high (54 ml/mm Hg right atrial pressure change in the patient just described) and the volume required therefore limited. Also maintenance of the right atrial pressure at the level indicated causes haemoconcentration by inducing a shift of fluid out of the circulating compartnent into the extracellular space, which is offset by the use of Dextran or plasma, which by their osmotic effect keep some of this fluid within the vascular compartment.

5.5. The dangers of pulmonary angiography

The radiographic contrast material required for the angiographic proof of pulmonary embolism produces systemic arterial vasodilatation. Following its injection it seems probable that the systemic venous bed also dilates; certainly the right atrial pressure falls rapidly without any known change in the circulating volume. The consequence of the fall in right atrial pressure is a diminution in right-sided stroke work, a net shift of blood out of the pulmonary bed into the systemic and a rise in the pulmonary vascular resistance. The inevitable fall in cardiac output may be to levels inadequate to sustain life. This chain of events is readily preventable if a short-acting α-agonist, phenylephrine, is administered immediately before the contrast material, in a dose sufficient to produce a measurable increase in systolic blood pressure (0·1–0·5 mg).

5.6. Inotropic stimulation

No evidence can be presented of the effect of inotropic stimulants in this situation, but adrenaline may be more advantageous than isoprenaline because of its α-stimulating effect upon the systemic venous capacity bed. If adrenaline is used the inspired oxygen tension must be kept high because the arterial oxygen tension is inevitably impaired in major pulmonary embolism.

5.7. The relevance of the pattern of circulatory disturbance to conventional therapy

The manoeuvres outlined above do not absolve the physician from the more generally accepted approaches to the treatment of pulmonary embolism. Many of these, apart from the administration of heparin in large doses, are of debated value, and indeed some such as morphine and diuretics are detrimental. Clearly, adjustment of the obstructed circulation to obtain optimal flows must be supported by efforts to prevent further embolism.

Both streptokinase[21] and urokinase have been shown to produce a short-term improvement in haemodynamics, including a decrease in pulmonary vascular resistance, but the advantage over the control groups, who were treated with heparin alone, disappeared after one week. It is not unreasonable to argue that some, at least, of the short-term improvement observed may have been due to the circulatory expansion and elevation of right atrial pressure which accompanied the administration of the thrombolytic agents. It is unfortunate that a control group was not treated with an equal volume of thrombolytically inert but otherwise similar material.

5.8. Acute lethal pulmonary embolism

If, in the presence of acute massive pulmonary embolism, the right atrial pressure is found to be of the order of 20 mm Hg spontaneously (without volume expansion), pulmonary embolectomy is indicated. Right atrial pressure elevation of this order is associated with critically low flows and is an indication for immediate intervention. Embolectomy has proved to be both possible and effective in this group.

It is neither possible nor appropriate to discover the equations of performance in this situation by measurement because such a circulation is unstable. It is possible to make certain deductions from such measurements as are available. In a patient with a right atrial pressure of 20 mm Hg, the measured mean pulmonary artery pressure was 30 mm Hg. A reasonable maximum estimate for the stroke volume is 20 ml/beat. These values produce a right-sided stroke work of 3 gram metres. This gives co-ordinates for a single point on the right-sided work equation of (20, < 3). Reference to Fig. 30 places a right heart with such co-ordinates amongst the most grossly disordered, with an equation $W_R = 0{\cdot}1\ P_R + 1$ or worse. Physiologically this means that the final disintegration of the circulation occurs with a well filled, dilated and near-inert right heart. After surgical removal of emboli, such hearts may require supportive cardiopulmonary bypass for some time before the overstretched right heart regains a more effective volume.

5.9. Chronic pulmonary embolism

A patient suffering from chronic packed pulmonary embolism, who was to be treated by inferior-vena-caval ligation, was investigated to establish what levels of right atrial pressure might be maintained with advantage following the ligation.

The equations of stroke volume (Fig. 42) show the same lateral transposition, which was observed acute pulmonary embolism. The venous tone is high (61 ml/mm Hg right atrial pressure change), and, with a 700 ml volume reduction produced by venesection, right atrial pressure falls from 19 to 7·5 mm Hg, the right-sided stroke work from 25 to 18 gram metres, and the pulmonary vascular resistance rises from 15 to 21 units. With the decrease in stroke work and rise in pulmonary vascular resistance, the stroke volume falls from 43 to 28 ml and the cardiac output from 3·9 to 2·6 l/min. The only apparent differences between the acute and chronic cases are the

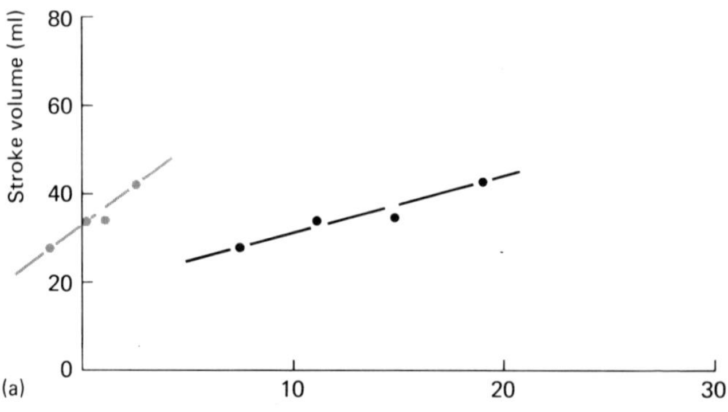

(a)

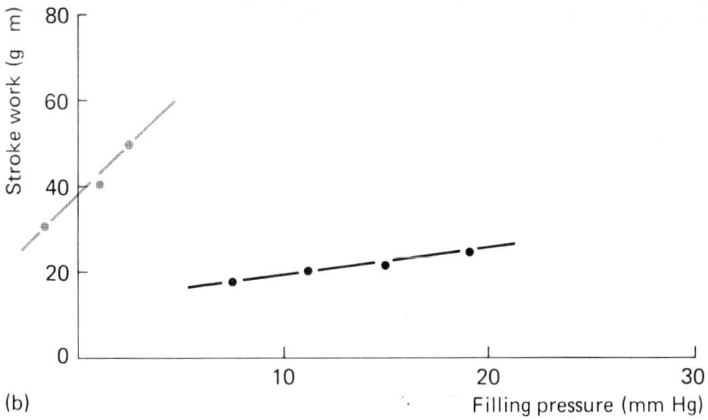

Fig. 42 The equations of (a) stroke volume and (b) stroke work in a case of chronic packed pulmonary embolism, showing the same configuration as was observed with acute pulmonary embolism.

higher values of right-sided stroke work and pulmonary resistance in the latter.

5.10. Ligation of the inferior vena cava

The findings are particularly cogent to inferior-vena-caval ligation, for the points of danger in such an operation become very clear. First, it is important not to use a myocardial depressant to induce anaesthesia. Figure 43 shows the disastrous effect of cyclopropane upon the right ventricular pressure record in these circumstances, and the restoration of the situation by external cardiac massage. Second, the right atrial pressure must be kept high in the face of any haemorrhage or the α-blocking effect of any anaesthetic agents. Third, and of vital importance, the right atrial pressure must be maintained at a very high level (between 10 and 15 mm Hg above the sternal angle in the case described in section 5·9) during the 36 hours following the ligation. During this period as much as 10 litres may be lost from the circulation into the extracellular space of the drainage area of the ligated inferior vena cava. The amount of this loss is unpredictable, but probably depends upon the extent to which the venous system is chronically occluded with thrombus. The fluid should be replaced as extracellular fluid, administered in such volume as is necessary to keep the right atrial pressure at the level described.

5.11. Chronic obstructive airways disease

If patients suffering from acute and chronic pulmonary embolism are made worse by treatment with diuretics but markedly improved by the maintenance of a high right atrial pressure, is the same true of

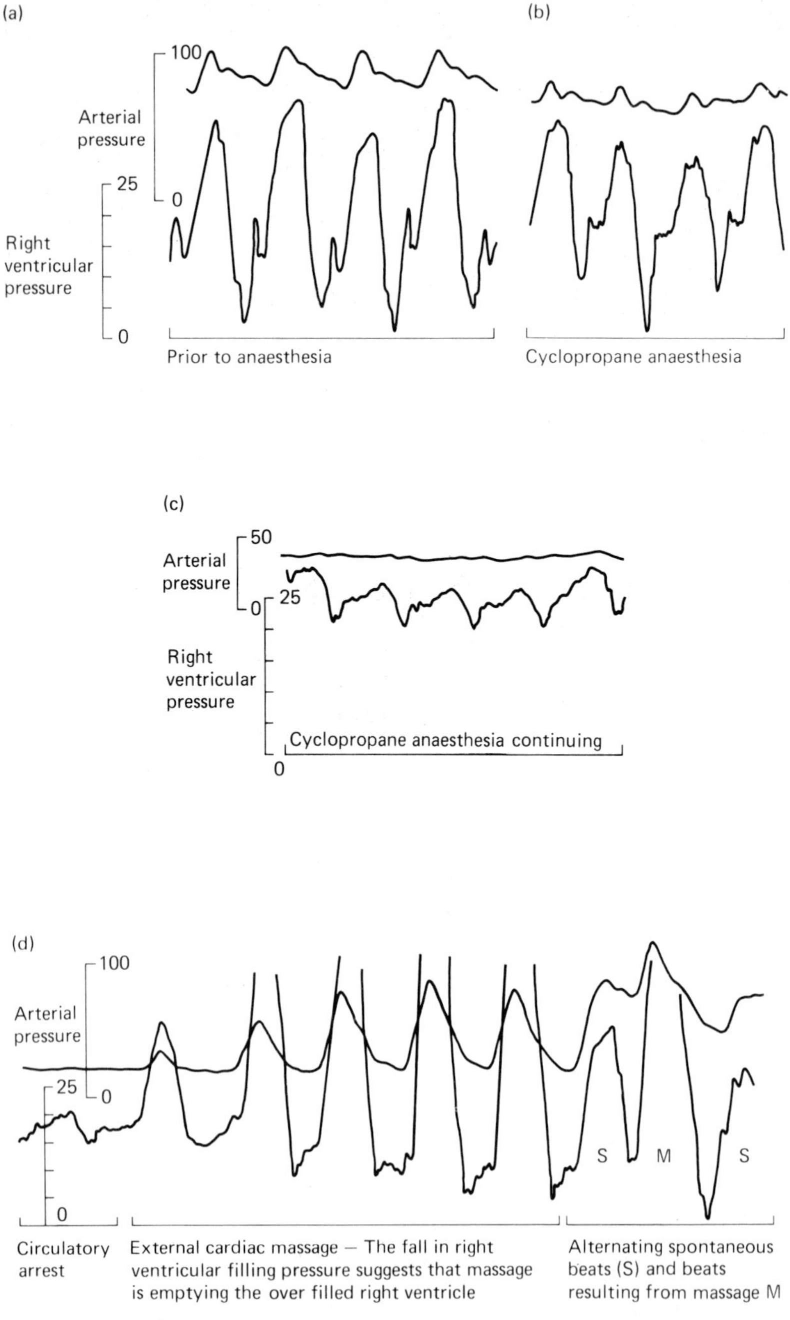
(a)
(b)
100
Arterial
pressure
25
0
Right
ventricular
pressure
0
Prior to anaesthesia
Cyclopropane anaesthesia
(c)
50
Arterial
pressure
0
25
Right
ventricular
pressure
Cyclopropane anaesthesia continuing
0
(d)
100
Arterial
pressure
25
0
S
M
S
0
Circulatory
arrest
External cardiac massage – The fall in right
ventricular filling pressure suggests that massage
is emptying the over filled right ventricle
Alternating spontaneous
beats (S) and beats
resulting from massage M

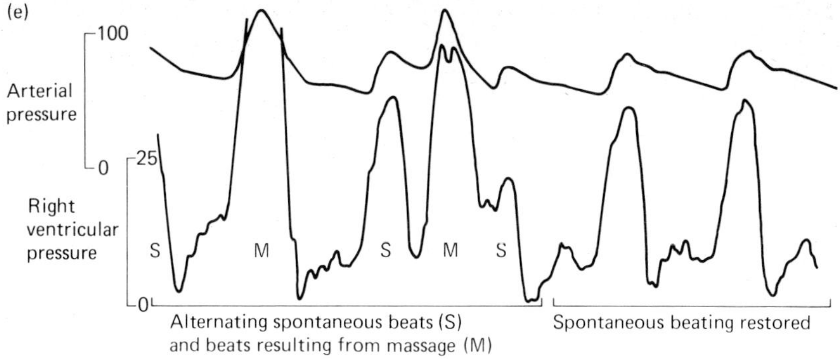

Fig. 43 (a)–(e) Record of the right ventricular pressure in a case of major pulmonary embolism, during induction of anaesthesia with cyclopropane, and subsequent restoration of the circulation by external cardiac massage.

patients with severe chronic obstructive airways disease? Both have 'cor pulmonale'; do they have the same pattern of circulatory derangement? The equations of stroke volume and stroke work in relation to filling pressure in a case of severe chronic bronchitis are shown in Figs. 44 and 45. Although the stroke volume equations are not

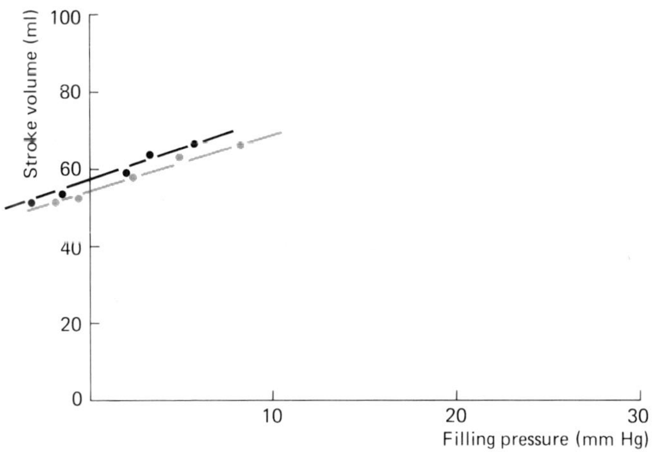

Fig. 44 Equations of stroke volume in a case of severe chronic bronchitis. Corresponding values of atrial pressure are close together due to the coincidence of a raised pulmonary vascular resistance (PVR 4 units) and a low systemic resistance (SVR 15 units), in the presence of normal stroke work equations (Fig. 45) for both sides of the heart. The important difference between this patient and the cases of pulmonary embolism is the very much higher values of stroke volume.

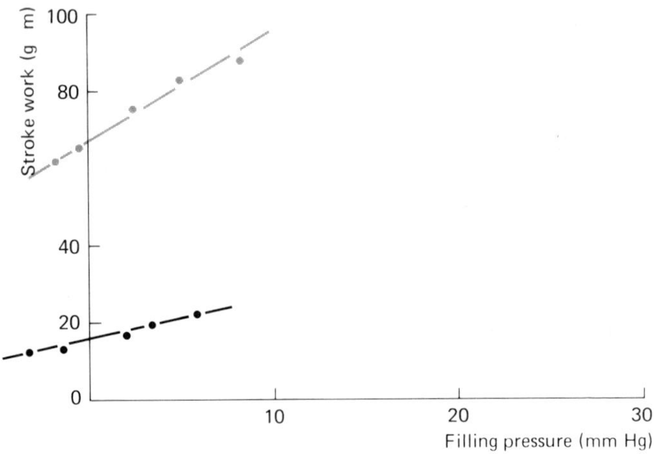

Fig. 45 The stroke work equations for both left and right heart of the patient with severe chronic bronchitis are within normal limits.

laterally transposed, as they were in the cases of pulmonary embolism they do lie abnormally close together. This configuration confirms that better flows can be obtained without risk of pulmonary oedema, by maintenance of high right atrial pressures.

5.12. What are the optimal circulatory conditions for the chronic bronchitic?

The vital requirement is to place the elements of dysfunction in their proper perspective. The critical problem in the patient whose circulation is obstructed with pulmonary emboli is a deficient cardiac output. This is not true of the patient with chronic obstructive airways disease, whose critical problem is deficient ventilation. The difference between a cardiac output of 6·5 l/min, which obtains with the spontaneously high right atrial pressure of 6 mm Hg and a figure of 5.5 l/min when the right atrial pressure is reduced to −3 mm Hg is of small account, for the patient's ventilation is worse at the higher filling pressures.

It may be argued, with some justification, that the information here presented is not representative of the naturally occurring disease state, since it was obtained under conditions of positive pressure ventilation with the arterial carbon dioxide tension maintained at the same level as had been achieved by spontaneous ventilation.

With the change of right atrial pressure from 5·8 to −3·2 mm Hg, the arterial CO_2 tension falls from 10·5 to 9·2 kPa (79 to 69 mm

Hg), the arterial O_2 tension rises from 8.0 to 9·6 kPa (60 to 72 mm Hg), the minute volume is unchanged at 6·2 l/min and the inflation pressure falls from 41 to 38 cm H_2O. The settings of the volume-cycled ventilator were not altered during this time.

The reasons for the improvement in ventilation at lower filling pressures are probably many, but two obvious possibilities are (1) the inevitable shift of blood from the pulmonary to the systemic circuit, producing greater pulmonary compliance, and (2) the effect of lowering the right atrial pressure upon the lymphatic drainage of the bronchial mucosa, which, if improved, might diminish airway obstruction.

5.13. Comparison of the circulatory findings in pulmonary embolism and chronic bronchitis

Although the fact that the bronchitic patient was artifically ventilated may, to some extent, vitiate the circulatory findings, there are some sharp contrasts with pulmonary embolic disease, which are probably disease dependent.

In addition to the very marked difference in cardiac output (6·3 l/min in contrast to 1·9 l/min at the same right atrial pressure), the venous tone in the chronic bronchitic, 161 ml/mm Hg right atrial pressure change, is very much less than the 54 and 61 ml/mm Hg change seen in the cases with pulmonary emboli, and the systemic vascular resistance is low, varying from 15 to 16 units as the equations were inscribed.

The physiological picture of the chronic bronchitic with relatively high flows, a low systemic vascular resistance and oedema is a familiar one. The contrast with the haemodynamics of pulmonary embolism with low flows, a high venous tone and a raised systemic vascular resistance may relate to differing degrees of water-salt retention. The venous pressure is raised in both conditions; it seems possible that a greater proportion of this rise may be due to water-salt retention and expansion of the circulating volume in chronic bronchitis, in contrast to an emphasis upon the high venous tone in pulmonary embolism.

6

Epilogue

6.1. Is cardiopulmonary bypass a disease entity?

It is common clinical experience that many of the patients undergoing heart surgery are treated intensively with diuretics prior to surgery, whereas following operation they undergo circulatory volume expansion upon a scale which may produce positive blood balances in excess of 1 litre.

The sudden circulatory change wrought by operation which makes volume expansion of benefit to the patient, could be due to an improvement in the function of the left heart or a decrease in venous tone occasioned by analgesic agents; there are other possibilities.

The stroke volume equations in Fig. 46 were inscribed following an aortic and mitral valve replacement, and show the apposition of the equations typical of the period following bypass surgery.[22] It is unusual for the atrial pressures to be separated by more than 8 mm Hg, whatever the lesion which has been corrected. It is for this reason that right atrial pressure values up to 10 mm Hg are tolerated without pulmonary oedema.

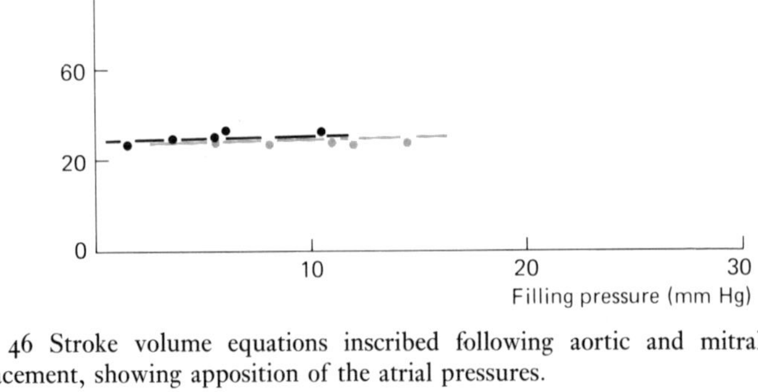

Fig. 46 Stroke volume equations inscribed following aortic and mitral valve replacement, showing apposition of the atrial pressures.

The stroke volume equations must always have a small positive slope, however bad the function, for reasons already explained (section 4.12), so that the best possible flows without pulmonary oedema will usually be obtained with a right atrial pressure between 5 and 10 mm Hg above the sternal angle.

It is important not to take the view that, if extremely abnormal hearts are best treated in this way postoperatively, then it must be safe to treat all hearts in this manner after any operation. Nothing could be further from the truth. It is cardiopulmonary bypass which produces these very special conditions, and the stroke work equations (Fig. 47) reveal what is almost certainly the principal factor involved. The right ventricular stroke work equations following

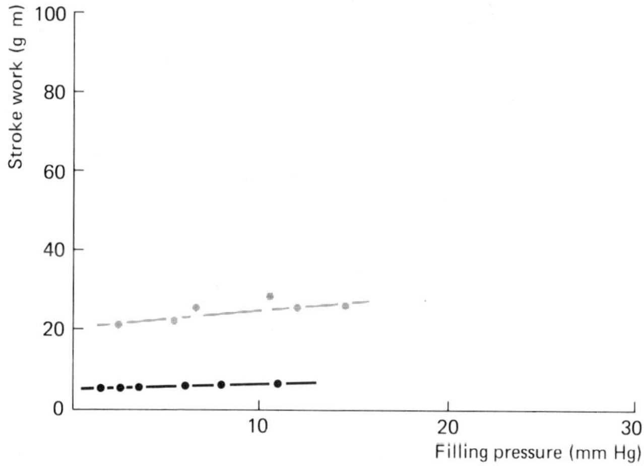

Fig. 47 Stroke work equations of the same case as Fig. 46, showing considerable impairment of the function of the right heart as well as the left.

bypass are remarkably flat, unless there has been pre-existing pulmonary hypertension.

On theoretical grounds the stroke volume equations could have been brought into this configuration by an improvement in function of the left side of the heart or a diminution in left ventricular afterload on the one hand, or an increase in right ventricular afterload or a deterioration in right ventricular function, on the other.

It is possible that all these factors may bear upon the matter, for aortic or mitral valve replacement ought to improve the function of the left heart, and analgesics are likely to diminish the left ventricular afterload. The circulating debris consequent upon the use of bypass could well raise the pulmonary vascular resistance. The remarkably low values of right ventricular stroke work observed in a variety of cardiopulmonary bypass cases suggest that right ventricular dysfunction is the principal factor.

The right ventricular dysfunction could be a purely local phenomenon, due to some peculiarity of bypass technique, but the almost universal experience concerning the optimal filling pressures after open heart surgery suggests that the pattern of apposed stroke volume equations is general.

6.2. The technology of treatment changes; the physiology of disease should be less evanescent

The equations of dysfunction, and the associated phenomena of venous tone, and vascular resistance in a number of circulatory states have been described. The description is not exhaustive, and the therapeutic suggestions which derive from the physiology are unlikely to be complete. Techniques for dealing with disease change very rapidly, but the mathematical statements about the principles of operation, if correct, should remain true.

Always the truth seems to lie in simplicity; the overtransfused patient is suffering from overtransfusion not heart failure, the acute nephritic cannot get rid of water, the patient with a pulmonary embolus has an obstructed circulation, the patient with chronic bronchitis is suffering from underventilation, and heart failure is better diagnosed from a clinical judgement that there is something amiss with the heart, than from the height of the venous pressure.

In the presence of heart failure, the dissociation of the problems of inadequate flows from those of pulmonary oedema will produce therapy better tailored to the patient's disease.

References

1. Sarnoff, S. J. and Berglund, E. (1954). Ventricular Function 1. Starling's law of the heart studied by means of simultaneous right and left ventricular function curves. *Circulation*, **9**, 706.
2. Guyton, A. C. and Lindsey, A. W. (1959). Effect of elevated left atrial pressure and decreased plasma protein concentration on the development of pulmonary oedema. *Circulation Research*, **7**, 649.
3. Fick, A. (1882). *Mechanische Arbeit und Warmeentwicklung bei der Muskelthatigheit*. F. A. Brackhaus, Leipzig.
4. Hill, A. V. (1938). The heat of shortening and the dynamic constants of muscle. *Proceedings of the Royal Society*, Series B, **126**, 136.
5. Roach, M. R. and Burton, A. C. (1957). The reason for the shape of the distensibility curves of arteries. *Canadian Journal of Biochemistry and Physiology*, **35**, 681.
6. Sonnenblick, E. H., Spiro, H. and Spiro, D. (1964). Role of the sarcomere in ventricular function and the mechanism of heart failure. *Circulation Research*, **15**, Supplement 2, 70.
7. Linzbach, A. J. (1960). Heart failure from the point of view of quantitative anatomy. *American Journal of Cardiology*, **5**, 370.
8. Woods, R. H. (1892). A few applications of a physical theorem to membrane in the human body in a state of tension. *Journal of Anatomy and Physiology*, **26**, 302.
9. Burton, A. C. (1957). The importance of the shape and size of the heart. *American Heart Journal*, **54**, 801.
10. Cohen, L. S., Wechsler, A. S., Mitchell, J. H. and Glick, G. (1970). Depression of cardiac function by streptomycin and other antimicrobial agents. *American Journal of Cardiology*, **26**, 505.
11. Sarnoff, S. J., Mitchell, J. H., Gilmore, J. P. and Remensnyder, P. (1960). Homeometric autoregulation in the heart. *Circulation Research*, **8**, 1077.
12. Branthwaite, M. A. and Bradley, R. D. (1968). Measurement of cardiac output by thermal dilution in man. *Journal of Applied Physiology*, **24**, 434.

13. Bradley, R. D., Jenkins, B. S. and Branthwaite, M. A. (1970). The influence of atrial pressure on cardiac performance following myocardial infarction complicated by shock. *Circulation*, **42**, 827.
14. Jenkins, B. S., Bradley, R. D. and Branthwaite, M. A. (1970). Evaluation of pulmonary arterial end diastolic pressure as an indirect estimate of left atrial mean pressure. *Circulation*, **42**, 75.
15. Bradley, R. D., Jenkins, B. S. and Branthwaite, M. A. (1971). Myocardial function in acute glomerulonephritis. *Cardiovascular Research*, **5**, 223.
16. Fishberg, A. M. (1937). *Heart Failure*. Henry Kimpton, London.
17. Maroko, P. R., Braunwald, E., Covell, J. W. and Ross, J. Jnr (1969). Factors influencing severity of myocardial ischaemia following experimental coronary occlusion. *Circulation*, **40**, Supplement 3, 140.
18. Mueller, H., Ayres, S. M., Gianelli, S., Conklin, E. F., Mazzara, J. T. and Grace, W. J. (1972). Effect of isoproterenol, l-norepinephrine and intra-aortic counterpulsation on haemodynamics and myocardial metabolism in shock following acute myocardial infarction. *Circulation*, **45**, 335.
19. Cohn, J. N., Guiha, N. H., Broder, M. I. and Limas, C. J. (1974). Right ventricular infarction. Clinical and haemodynamic features. *American Journal of Cardiology*, **33**, 209.
20. Cohn, J. N., Tristani, F. E. and Khatri, I. M. (1969). Studies in clinical shock and hypotension. VI. Relationship between left and right ventricular function. *Journal of Clinical Investigation*, **48**, 2008.
21. Miller, G. A. H., Sutton, G. C., Kerr, I. H., Gibson, R. V. and Honey, M. (1971). Comparison of streptokinase and heparin in treatment of isolated acute massive pulmonary embolism. *British Medical Journal* **ii**, 681.
22. Jenkins, B. S., Branthwaite, M. A. and Bradley, R. D. (1973). Cardiac function after open heart surgery. *Cardiovascular Research*, **7**, 297.

Index